QP

23 1080790 2

The Henry E. Sigerist Supplements to the
Bulletin of the History of Medicine
New Series, no. 2
Editor: Lloyd G. Stevenson

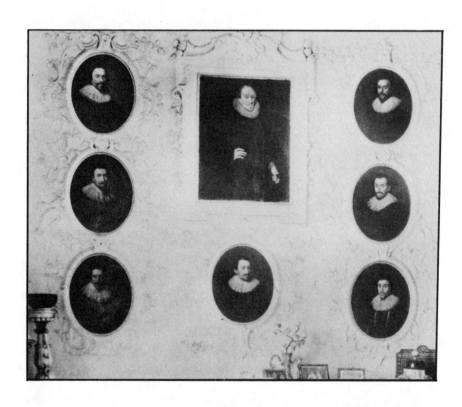

Portraits of William Harvey (upper right) and his six brothers, surrounding that of their father, Thomas. The latter was a self-made businessman, and all the sons except William and John (middle left) were overseas merchants in the City of London. The group is shown here as it once hung in the music room at Rolls Park, in Essex, a house that belonged to the family of Eliab Harvey (upper left) but is no longer extant. (From photograph in the collection of the Institute of the History of Medicine, The Johns Hopkins University.)

WILLIAM HARVEY AND HIS AGE

The Professional and Social Context of the Discovery of the Circulation

Edited by
Jerome J. Bylebyl

The Johns Hopkins University Press • Baltimore and London

Manufactured in the United States of America

The Johns Hopkins University Press, Baltimore, Maryland 21218
The Johns Hopkins Press Ltd., London

Library of Congress Catalog Number 78-20526
ISBN 0-8018-2213-0

Library of Congress Cataloging in Publication Data
Main entry under title:

William Harvey and his age.

(The Henry E. Sigerist supplements to the Bulletin
of the history of medicine; new ser., no. 2)
Papers from a conference held in Kansas City, May 13,
1978, sponsored by the American Association for the
History of Medicine.
Includes bibliographical references and index.
1. Harvey, William, 1578-1657.   2. Blood—Circula-
tion—History—Congresses.   3. Physiologists—England
—Biography.   4. Physicians—England—Biography.
I. Bylebyl, Jerome J.   II. American Association for
the History of Medicine.   III. Series.
QP26.H3W544   612'.1'0924 [B]   78-20526
ISBN 0-8018-2213-0

CONTENTS

Preface

Nineteen seventy-eight has been a year for celebrating the life and accomplishments of William Harvey because it is the 350th anniversary of his publication of the discovery of the circulation of the blood and the 400th anniversary of his birth. The present volume grew out of one such celebration, held at Kansas City on May 13, 1978, as part of the annual meeting of the American Association for the History of Medicine. However, all three essays are based upon longstanding researches into Harvey's work and influence, and so are not just occasional pieces in the usual sense. Moreover, without much prior consultation it turned out that there was a major theme common to all three papers, that of the interaction between Harvey's scientific achievement and his professional identity as a practicing physician. Hence, it seemed especially appropriate to arrange for this joint publication of the three essays, which have been revised in varying degrees from the papers originally read.

As a scientist Harvey was of course *sui generis,* but he chiefly made his way in his society by filling a decidedly more conventional role, that of the elite, classically educated physician. This meant that his biological investigations were necessarily interspersed with various professional activities, including notably the treatment and advising of individual patients, and involvement in the corporate affairs of the London College of Physicians, the professional body to which he belonged. Moreover, one does not have to look very far to find some obvious connections between Harvey's scientific and professional activities. For example, on the title page of *De motu cordis* he identified himself as "Professor of Anatomy at the College of Physicians of London," and in the dedication to the President and Fellows of the College he made it clear that his official College lectures had provided an important forum for the development and testing of his ideas about the movement of the heart and blood. Again, his physiological writings are replete with observations drawn from his experience with human patients, as well as with theoretical discussions of disease and its treatment.

The three essays in this volume address themselves to various aspects of this complex interaction between Harvey's anatomical and physiological investigations and his role as a physician. Charles Webster considers how the distinctive characteristics of Jacobean London and the status of medicine within that society may have affected the general scientific outlook and particular interests of a physician like Harvey. He portrays a city facing massive health problems, and a learned medical profession whose position was rather precarious, in part because of its inadequacy in meeting those problems. He suggests that this crisis created a climate that was quite conducive to innovative thinking by physicians and others concerned with natural philosophy, and shows how a number of the themes in Harvey's biological investigations had their counterparts in the broader intellectual currents of his city.

My own essay also considers the professional medical context of the discovery of the circulation, but in a different sense. My focus is not on the unique features of medicine in Harvey's London, but rather on the attitudes toward disease and its treatment that were common to all physicians educated in the classical tradition. I argue that in this tradition no sharp distinction could be made between normal physiological processes, on the one hand, and the abnormal effects of disease and therapy, on the other. And I try to show that there are many ways in which attention to pathological and therapeutic issues can help us to understand both the difficulty of arriving at a conception of the circulation, and how that realization was finally achieved.

Robert Frank reverses the polarity of the first two essays to consider what effect Harvey's discoveries had upon his own professional reputation, the activities of his fellow physicians, and the status of the medical profession within English society. He notes that in the early seventeenth century Harvey was unique among the collegiate physicians of London in his dedication to original anatomical research, and that for some time after 1628 his theory of circulation was met with aloofness by his colleagues and suspicion by some of his patients. By the 1650s, however, all of this had dramatically changed, for not only had the circulation gained wide acceptance both at home and abroad, but, as Frank illustrates in detail, Harvey came into his own as the archetype of a whole group of English physicians who greatly enhanced the status of their profession precisely through their original anatomical researches.

The three essays do not, of course, exhaust the theme of how Harvey's investigations were affected by and in turn affected the professional and social context in which they were carried out. However, it is hoped that they will serve to delineate some of the important aspects of this interaction, as well as to stimulate the consideration of additional ones. And perhaps they may also help to illuminate some broader issues, such as the motivation to basic medical research, its relationship to clinical practice, and its effect on the perception of the medical professional by those outside its ranks.

On behalf of all three authors, I should like to express appreciation to Ronald Numbers, the Chairman of the Program Committee of the AAHM, who first suggested the Harvey symposium and contributed much to its planning; to Robert Hudson, the Local Arrangements Chairman, for his unfailing cooperation, and especially for obtaining the support from the University of Kansas which made it possible for Charles Webster to join our proceedings; and to Saul Jarcho, who introduced and chaired the session with grace and skill. Our warm thanks are also due to the Council of the AAHM for generously agreeing to subsidize this special supplement to the *Bulletin of the History of Medicine;* to John Blake, David Cowen, and Barbara Rosenkrantz, the Editorial Committee of the Association, for their prompt consideration of the manuscript; and to Michael Aronson and Anders Richter of The Johns Hopkins University Press, who helped smooth the path toward its early publication.

I must also say a special word of gratitude to Lloyd Stevenson and Janet Koudelka, my colleagues at the Johns Hopkins Institute of the History of Medicine. It was Dr. Stevenson's initiative that led to the decision to publish these three essays as a separate volume, and he has been a steady source of assistance and encouragement in the realization of the plan. And Mrs. Koudelka, despite her many other duties, undertook the copy editing of the manuscript, a task that she has carried out with her customary thoroughness and care. Finally, I am greatly indebted to my secretary, Mrs. Mary Moore, who (apart from endless retyping of my own essay) has helped so much in the arrangement of the original symposium and in preparing this volume for the press.

Introduction

Saul Jarcho

William Harvey, author of *De motu cordis,* is far more than a venerated idol surrounded by chanting acolytes, nor is he an antique mummy, stuffed with obligatory or perfunctory panegyrics. He is a live historical personage, the subject of vigorous debate. This fact is evident in the researches and writings of the three scholars who here set before you the results of their reflections. It is evident also in the voluminous writings of Dr. Walter Pagel and in the less copious but nevertheless highly important contributions of Mrs. Gweneth Whitteridge. The former has given us an elaborate, fundamental, philosophical, and Germanic portrayal; the latter has offered us a realistic British depiction; and it is hard to tell whether the differences between the two can be resolved by additional research or must remain forever in the more subjective realms of literary, personal, and national tastes.

We justly venerate Harvey as a clinical experimenter and discoverer, but in doing so we employ the foreshortening and compression that we usually inflict on persons whose lives and work we attempt to summarize. It is well known that Harvey was not only an experimenter but also an Aristotelian. He was, in addition, a Virgilian. And, as Mrs. Whitteridge has pointed out, in his work on locomotion (*De motu locali animalium*) he was not an experimenter but a scholastic—i.e., a compiler and weighmaster of inherited doctrines.

While this description of Harvey's early myologic treatise is correct as far as it goes, it does not do justice to the difficulties, since in that phase of his researches Harvey was attempting to explain the action of muscles, but the fundamental facts of chemistry and histology had not yet been discovered. In other words, he had chosen a problem but the elements necessary for its solution did not then exist.

Incidental considerations of this kind do nothing to detract from Harvey's fame but merely point to some of the complexities and tell us in advance that there is much to be discussed by the authors of this book. Chauncey Leake's translation of *De motu cordis,* first published in 1928, has passed through five editions. This in itself is clear evidence of Harvey's vitality. So also, and almost thirty years later, is the Italian translation by Loris Premuda. Most recent of translations is the English text of Mrs. Whitteridge.

In addition to these and other translations there have appeared in recent years many studies and interpretations of Harvey's work, which will be found listed in the documentation of the papers that follow. The pursuit has even extended all the way to entomology, although medical interest has not been carried so far. Medical historians, as specialized as other scholars, regularly overlook the fact that William Harvey founded the cardiology of insects. This fact, recognized by entomologists such as J. C. Jones,[1] is evident in the *De motu cordis* chapter IV, where Harvey says (in Leake's translation): "Even in wasps, hornets, and flies, have I seen with a lens a beating heart at the upper part of what is called tail." This observation, like other Harveian discoveries, was later developed by Malpighi.

We are thankful to Dr. Robert Hudson and to the University of Kansas for making possible Dr. Charles Webster's recent visit to the United States. Dr. Webster is Reader in the History of Medicine at Oxford University and Fellow of Corpus Christi College. When I proclaim that we have been honored by his visit, such announcement rests *inter alia* on his massive and magisterial treatise *The Great Instauration,* a study "of the scientific, medical and social ideas of the English Puritans." This work, replete with thoughtful discussions of medicine, necessarily includes much discussion of William Harvey. In the present book Dr. Webster writes on "William Harvey and the Crisis of Medicine in Jacobean England."

The editor of this volume, Dr. Jerome J. Bylebyl, is Assistant Professor at the Institute of the History of Medicine and holds the same appointment in the Department of the History of Science at Johns Hopkins University. His doctoral thesis dealt with cardiovascular physiology in the sixteenth and early seventeenth centuries. His more recent writings have examined this subject and its congeners in detail and have also been concerned with Galenic physiology. Many will have read and admired the biography of Harvey which Dr. Bylebyl contributed to the *Dictionary of Scientific Biography* (VI. 150–162). His contribution to the present volume is titled "The Medical Side of Harvey's Discovery: The Normal and the Abnormal."

Dr. Robert G. Frank is a member of the Medical History Division of the Department of Anatomy at UCLA. He is fortunate in combining knowledge of zoology and knowledge of history. His research on seventeenth-century English anatomy and physiology and his studies of the Oxford Harveians form an appropriate background for the paper with which he favors us here. It is titled "The Physician-Scientist as Hero: The Image of Harvey in Restoration England."

*Jack C. Jones. *The Circulatory System of Insects* (Springfield: Thomas, 1977), p. vii.

William Harvey and His Age

William Harvey and
the Crisis of Medicine in Jacobean England

Charles Webster

William Harvey's "vegetative" existence as a conventional London and court physician seems to be altogether less interesting, and almost disso- ciated from, his brilliant investigations in the field of experimental biology. The impetus for Harvey's scientific work seems to have been provided more by the writings that stemmed from the Renaissance anatomical tradition, than by the relatively undistinguished medical culture of Jacobean London. This present essay reappraises Harvey's career, with a view to suggesting that there was not a complete divorce between scientific and professional preoccu- pations. In this context it is particularly relevant that Harvey's biological ideas were framed at a time when London was experiencing a major crisis of health, and when there was deep conflict within the ranks of its medical prac- titioners. This situation generated destructive professional rivalries; it also provided a climate congenial to debate, diversification, and innovation in the fields of medicine and natural philosophy. Harvey's scientific work may be regarded as one of the most important ingredients in this pattern of events. In the same context it is notable that, although most of Harvey's published work appeared after 1648, the bulk of his scientific investigations and writing took place before that date, and indeed before the outbreak of the Civil War. The text of his *Praelectiones* dates mainly from before 1620; *De motu cordis* from before 1628; *De generatione* was largely completed by 1640, and it may have been largely researched and written by 1636.

It is accepted that in the late sixteenth century London became one of the most rapidly expanding urban centers in Europe. By 1600 its population had reached 200,000.[1] In the course of the seventeenth century the rise in population continued unabated, until by 1700 London was the largest city in Europe. At the time of Harvey's death London housed no less than 7 percent of England's population. The size of London and the density of its popula- tion amazed contemporary observers. In 1600 no other English town pos- sessed a population of more than 15,000. The escalating problems of disease facing London's burgeoning population can easily be imagined. London ex-

perienced a major outbreak of plague in 1603, shortly after Harvey's return
to England from Padua. Harvey was one of the physicians deputed by the
College to advise the city authorities about the plague epidemics of 1625 and
1630. The epidemics of 1603 and 1625 were major social and demographical
catastrophes, between them claiming more than 80,000 victims.[2] Sporadic
plague epidemics were merely the most spectacular features of a scene that
was marked by a general and alarmingly high level of mortality and mor-
bidity. Evidence from all sources testifies to the great anxiety about health at
all levels in the population in the first half of the seventeenth century. The
Bills of Mortality issued on a weekly basis were apprehensively scrutinized for
signs of the ebb and flow of diseases.[3] The city that at one moment was so
teeming that its streets seemed to be "paved with men," at the time of infec-
tion became so deserted that they seemed to be turning instead into herb
gardens.[4]

Disease periodically disrupted the economic life of the capital, drove its
population into the countryside, emptied its churches, caused the court to
evacuate from London, and even threatened to effect an irrevocable breakdown in the corporate activities of the College of Physicians. Worst of all,
epidemics were associated in the minds of civic authorities with mass hysteria
and the breakdown of civil order.[5] Families, long used to a high level of infant mortality, became accustomed to experience the premature loss of their
dearest kin. The royal family was not immune to this depredation. The death
of the brilliant eighteen-year-old Prince Henry in 1612 was a cause for public
lamentations. In a similar context, Donne declared, "There is no health...
can there be worse sickness, than to know/That we are never well, nor can be
so?" Donne characterized a common mood of fatalistic pessimism in con-
cluding, "With new diseases on ourselves we war,/And with new physic, a
worse engine far."[6]

Such was the crisis of health at the time when William Harvey was establishing himself as a member of the College of Physicians of London. Problems of this kind were of course not new to physicians and civic authorities in
European towns and cities. Elaborate public health mechanisms had long
been in operation in Italian towns. If not entirely successful, they served to
preserve civic order and morale.[7] The large size and rapid expansion of London at once increased the scale of the public health problem, without introducing factors facilitating the institution of adequate public health
measures. The public health system of London was never more than a feeble
imitation of the continental model. The College of Physicians was conspicuously less active in public health affairs than its continental counterparts. In-

deed the College was in many respects a less successful organization than would have been expected from the auspicious circumstances of its foundation. Thomas Linacre and the humanistic founders and patrons gave every impression that the College would cultivate high standards of civic duty among physicians. Their model was More's *Utopia*, a work that displayed great sensitivity to the public health needs of urban communities.[8] Despite the genuine intellectual distinction of such figures as Linacre, Caius, and Gilbert, even by the time of Harvey's candidature the College had failed to secure a dominant and prestigious position among the civic institutions of London. As an extra-municipal corporation the College was not as well entrenched within the City as the Barber-Surgeons' Company and the Grocers' Company, and it never enjoyed more than indifferent relations with the civic authorities. Hence the physicians were little consulted at the time of public health emergencies, even when joint action was requested by the King and the Privy Council.

However, upon the request of the Lord Mayor, a committee comprising Harvey and three colleagues from the College of Physicians at least held a meeting with aldermen at the outset of the 1625 epidemic.[9] With the appearance of a new epidemic in 1629 the College, reluctantly responding to pressure from the King, held somewhat inconsequential discussions about providing plague physicians, and submitted a report on the likely causes for the spread of contagion.[10] A clue to the unwillingness of the College to participate more actively may be found in Harvey's complaint that during the 1625 epidemic the civic authorities had ignored the directions set down by the College representatives, and failed to support its physicians, having employed others instead. With respect to the latter Harvey specifically mentioned "Dr Anthony" and a Spaniard. According to civic records, a "Spanish doctor" and the surgeon Nicholas Heath were officially employed on plague relief. The writer and physician Thomas Lodge was also involved in this work.[11] In 1625 the city spent substantial sums of money on medical relief. Significantly none of the practitioners employed was at the time licensed by the College.

Not only was the College of little assistance in framing a more positive and sustained public health program, but it was a common cause for comment in 1603 as in 1665 that the elite among the physicians deserted London at the first appearance of epidemics. As Dekker wryly commented, "Never let any man ask one what became of our Physitions in this Massacre, they hid their Synodicall heads as well as the prowdest."[12] Apart from non-collegiate physicians like Thomas Lodge and Raphael Thorius, both of whom died during the 1625 plague, the population was largely dependent upon surgeons, apothecaries, and "Empiricall mad-caps" and "jolly Montebanks" who "clapt up their bills upon every post." In desperation the population consumed large quantities of such panaceas as Dragon Water and Mithridatum.[13]

The limited part played by the College in public health work is symptomatic of its general problem of coming to terms with the changing medical needs of a large urban population. Thus there was a danger of the College's lapsing into isolation and estrangement. Indeed the College made remarkably few concessions to changing conditions. The original structure of the College was scrupulously preserved; modifications to the statutes were rarely of more than technical relevance. Above all the College was resistant to increasing the size of its fellowship, or even expanding the number of candidates permitted at any one time. Thus the College between 1590 and 1640 preserved a membership of thirty (this number before 1618 excluding, after that date including, the royal physicians) and for most of this period there were a maximum of six candidates. It was intended that all others eligible to serve as physicians would register as licentiates, and thereby become eligible to pay not insubstantial annual fees. The College enjoyed a statutory right of supervision with respect to ancillary grades within the medical profession. In general, surgeons belonging to the Barber-Surgeons' Company, and apothecaries (associated with the Grocers' Company until 1617 and as a separate society after that date) were left to manage their own affairs, providing that they were careful not to trespass into the areas of practice preserved for physicians. The College regarded as a major responsibility the prevention of any intrusion into the practice of medicine by those lacking its authorization.

From the outset the College was presented with a major problem of enforcement of its wide legal powers over the control of the practice of medicine in the prescribed area of the city of London and its environs to an extent of seven miles. The College remained a vigorous force in London largely by virtue of its determination to preserve its monopoly over the practice of internal medicine, rather than by the positive role that its members played in the treatment of the ailments of London's sickly population.

The task that the College set itself was formidable, and ultimately almost all-engrossing. Between 1600 and 1640 the official records of the College are preoccupied with interminable disputes with sister medical organizations, and with the diverse classes of unorganized practitioners labeled by the College as illiterate "empirics." Very little of the business transacted by the College was unrelated to the above disputes. In this contest the College tended to overestimate its own ability to deploy the legal machinery available for restraining those guilty of delinquency. It also failed to take into account the degree of support that could be mobilized by its adversaries. Thus controls that Colleges of Physicians in Italian towns were able to employ to preserve their authority, proved to be impracticable in the London context.

It is a reflection of the relative weakness of the London College that only a handful of physicians came forward to register voluntarily as licentiates, and only a few others could be coerced into taking out licenses and paying regular fees. In addition surgeons and apothecaries occupied an entrenched position in the framework of city companies, and from a position of wealth and influence they increasingly trespassed into the practice of internal medicine. Outside the London companies hordes of unauthorized medical practitioners recruited from every social class, and every nationality of immigrant, openly breached the monopoly of the collegiate physicians. Thus even in the fifty years ending in 1600, for which records are seriously incomplete, the College had taken action against 236 unlicensed practitioners. In a large number of cases the result had been inconclusive or positively unfavorable to the College. Harvey entered the College at a time when the problem was escalating still further, but when, under a new monarch, empirics were being prosecuted with renewed vigor. Actions were brought against 435 individuals between 1601 and 1640. During the decades before 1640 Harvey was frequently directly drawn into proceedings against delinquents. Most of the Comitia attended by him were dominated by this issue. To Harvey and his colleagues the survival of the College, and the maintenance of essential academic and ethical standards in medicine, depended on the success of this enterprise. It was realized that failure on a variety of fronts was irrevocably damaging the standing of the College. At the end of the plague epidemic of 1625 Theodore Diodati (father of Milton's friend and correspondent Charles Diodati) complained that while he had dutifully paid regular fees, "empeiriques, ignorants practise and not paye."[14] Indeed he wanted to know by what rights a College that was "crusht and dasht" was continuing to demand fees from its licentiates. The mounting assaults of Diodati and others against the College in the decades before 1640 are reminiscent of Milton's own crushing indictment of monopolies in *Areopagitica*: "Truth and understanding are not such wares as to be monopolised and traded by tickets and statutes, and standards."[15] By the time of this statement the Civil War had begun, and all monopolies, including that exercised by the College, had been swept away.

The above outcome could not have been anticipated by William Harvey when his name was entered as a candidate at the College in 1603. At a small meeting of the President and senior members, Harvey was examined and his answers found satisfactory.[16] Even such an acceptable candidate as Harvey felt the burden of the complex rules of the College. Harvey was examined on two further occasions; he then awaited formal admission as a candidate. It took a year and a half for him to be given permission to practice, and he was to wait three years more before becoming eligible for a fellowship.[17] Under the College statutes Harvey, as an M.D. of Padua, having not undertaken the full seven years of arts studies leading to an M.A. at Cambridge, having not incorporated his medical degree at an English university, and having not become licensed by the College of Physicians upon his return to England, was liable not only to pay higher fees upon his admission, but also to be passed over in favor of candidates with different credentials. For instance, Edward Elwyn, a young Cambridge M.D. and licentiate, was examined for the first time on the occasion of Harvey's third examination, admitted as a candidate at the same time as Harvey, and elected to a fellowship eighteen months before Harvey.[18]

The struggle for precedence among candidates was a divisive factor in the College. The rules of admission were the subject of protracted debate at the time of Harvey's election, and on subsequent occasions. Even more divisive within the medical profession were those rules that precluded highly qualified foreigners from becoming more than licentiates, or the seemingly arbitrary disqualification of well-educated English physicians. Perhaps the roots of the antagonism of James Primerose toward the theory of circulation may be found in events surrounding his unsuccessful candidature in December and January 1629–30. Primerose, qualified with a Montpellier M.D. and having powerful court backing in his application for a fellowship, was even suggested by his patrons as a public lecturer in medicine. Primerose was of Scottish-French extraction; although initially treated favorably, he was later disqualified from candidature and the College placed every obstacle in the way of the lectureship. It is not surprising that the disgruntled Primerose, reflecting on the praise lavished on Harvey and his discovery at the Extraordinary Anatomical Lectures delivered in December 1629, should promptly embark on a savage attack on the distinguished innovator, and senior official of the College.[19]

Although granted a license at a cost of £8 plus the payment of various fees, Primerose retired from London to practice in Hull. Others treated less favorably include the well-known writer Thomas Lodge, an M.D. of Avignon who was examined along with Harvey and was found partly unsatisfactory.[20]

As already indicated, Lodge was already practicing medicine and he continued to practice successfully but illegally until his death during the 1625 plague epidemic. During the meetings that Harvey attended in the years following his election, he would have gained an impression of the scale of the problem of unlicensed practice and become introduced to leading and persistent adversaries of the College such as Thomas Bonham, Stephen Bredwell, John Burgess, and Peter Chamberlen, father and son, all of whom could call upon support from courtiers and aristocrats in their dealings with the College.

Harvey was brought into closer relationship with problems of discipline when he was appointed censor in Michaelmas 1613. The Annals of the College show that meetings were held with ever-increasing frequency during the first decade of the century. At one time quarterly Comitia had been sufficient. In the year of Harvey's censorship, meetings were often held at weekly intervals, largely in response to the problem of empirics. So pressing was this danger that the college appointed an influential committee, which included Harvey, to consider means of mobilizing support at court, in Parliament, and in law, for measures to suppress empirics. It was tersely commented that the disease was swelling—*Nam turget morbi materia.*[21]

Harvey and his three fellow censors dealt with a representative spectrum of unlicensed practitioners during the session 1613–14. Recorded actions were brought against twenty-six practitioners, and many other more minor breaches of College rules were dealt with. The largest identifiable groups of delinquents were the six apothecaries and five surgeons. Apothecaries were usually charged with dispensing medicines without prescriptions, and surgeons with trespassing into the practice of internal medicine. The most persistent and ambitious offender during Harvey's first term as censor was the surgeon Peter Chamberlen the younger, who appeared at the College to defend his "complex, ill and illicit practice." Chamberlen was to emerge as one of the most effective adversaries of the College.[22]

Impressions given by the College about the illiteracy and professional incompetence of unlicensed practitioners are not supported by the sample from 1613–14, or by evidence from other decades. No fewer than eight of the practitioners censured by Harvey and his colleagues were Englishmen who were university educated, and most of these possessed medical degrees. The most celebrated figures in this category were Francis Anthony and James Forester, both graduates of Cambridge, who had been constantly under harassment by the College for some time, and who were to continue in practice until the 1620s. Making his first appearance before the College in Harvey's year of office was Nicholas Fiske of Cambridge, who was establishing himself as London's leading astrological practitioner.[23] Of the two alien practitioners facing Harvey, one, John Tenant, possessed a Paris M.D.[24] The only category of illegal practitioner coming to Harvey's attention that can be assumed to have lacked formal education was the small group of three women practitioners. From the evidence brought against them they seem to have followed the normal course of specializing in the diseases of women and children. The appearance of women in the records is interesting as reflecting the prominent part played by women in popular medicine, and for confirming the determination of the College to stamp out even the most minor abuses of its privileges. Accordingly Susan Fletcher was warned to desist from her practice that consisted primarily of treating sore breasts with a lotion comprising milk, white bread, and herbs.[25]

Harvey's year of office as censor marked the beginning of certain major policy initiatives with respect to the control of subsidiary groups within the medical profession. One means explored to secure better discipline of inferior groups was that of encouraging a more formalized division of labor. Harvey was present at meetings called to discuss the establishment of a midwives' corporation. Initially the Fellows favored this proposal, particularly if licenses were to be granted to midwives only after their examination by the College. They undoubtedly hoped that this corporation might not only improve the current "very ignorant" practice of midwifery, but also provide means for the suppression of medical practice by women. The scheme collapsed when it became evident that the Chamberlen family were involved and were aiming to superintend the new corporation.[26]

A more important problem was presented by the activities of the apothecaries. The College had experienced little success in controlling the practices of apothecaries associated with the powerful Grocers' Company. In 1614 after discussions with the King it was decided that support should be given to the secession of apothecaries from the Grocers' Company.[27] It was felt that such an action would primarily be to the advantage of the College. A separate and well-regulated Society of Apothecaries would secure high status in return for the correction of their errors.[28] Harvey was one of the College majority supporting this course of action. He joined a committee charged with the compilation from existing handbooks of a dispensatory or pharmacopoeia which would be kept in the shops of apothecaries and would be vital for controlling their practice.[29] Harvey attended many of the subsequent discussions relating to the apothecaries and the pharmacopoeia. The formal separation of the Society of Apothecaries took place in December 1617 only after a long legal dispute with the Grocers who were, to the embarrassment of the College, supported by the eminent physician Sir William Paddy.[30] These disputes impinged on arrangements for the preparation of the pharmacopoeia, and they resulted in the humiliation of the withdrawal of the first issue and its replacement by a greatly revised edition in 1618.[31]

Any short-term advantage to the College through alliance with the apothecaries was offset by the intransigence of the Apothecaries' Society once its position was consolidated. Indeed from 1624 onwards both surgeons and apothecaries mounted a vigorous campaign at a parliamentary and popular level for the extension of their rights. Between then and the outbreak of the Civil War no effective means of containing them was devised by the College.

Harvey was present at meetings in June and July 1624 called to consider the abuses of surgeons and apothecaries. A committee comprising Harvey and five colleagues was formed to deliberate on the reform of the apothecaries.[32] But leading London apothecaries continued audaciously and persistently to breach the College's nominal monopoly of medical practice. Apothecaries insisted on an unrestricted right to retail any commodity falling within the purview of their trade. Apothecaries and physicians consequently became locked in a dispute that resulted in petitioning and counter-petitioning to the Privy Council and Attorney-General, and involved protracted actions in the Court of Exchequer and ultimately before the Star Chamber. No definitive conclusion had been reached by the beginning of the Civil War.

Harvey, as a senior figure within the College, was inevitably drawn into these conflicts. On behalf of the College he presented to the Privy Council a detailed set of proposals for the better control of apothecaries and surgeons.[33] In response to the College's accusation that apothecaries were guilty of the unscrupulous exploitation of dangerous drugs, the Apothecaries' Society filed a complaint that it was physicians who were guilty of dangerous practices, and they specifically accused William Harvey of being responsible for the death of a patient at St. Bartholomew's Hospital.[34] The College was obliged to investigate this charge. Harvey was of course cleared of blame by his colleagues. But the episode could have caused embarrassment, as did the almost simultaneous attack mounted on his colleague Robert Fludd, who was aggressively charged by William Foster with dabbling in magic and witchcraft in the course of his weapon-salve therapy. In his voluminous reply, Fludd speculated that his critic, a Buckinghamshire clergyman, was making trouble on behalf of the Barber-Surgeons' Company.[35]

Harvey was to make two further interventions in the dispute with the Apothecaries. Firstly, at a meeting between the disputing parties he was delegated to make a speech outlining the grounds upon which the College demanded conformity of the apothecaries.[36] Later, after his continental journey with the Earl of Arundel, he came forward to testify before the Star Chamber on the basis of his recent extensive experience of continental practices: "That in all places where he hath travelled As at Cullon, Frankford, Noremberg, Vyenna, Prage, Venice, Sienna, fflorence, Rome, Naples, the Apothecaries are in deference & dependency upon the Physicians, and for the most part tyed by oathes to certaine orders (as in ffrance is expressed by Renadeus in his dispensatory) their numbers lymitted, their medecines taxed, & tyed to make only such medicines for common sale as are appointed by the dispensatoryes of every severall place; And their Medecines searched & corrected by the physicians in all places."[37] Harvey's testimony was corroborated by the physicians Simon Baskerville and Ottowell Meverall, but vigorously denied by the Apothecaries' spokesman Gideon de Laune.

The above instances by no means exhaust the part played by Harvey in the service of the College of Physicians during the period of crisis in its affairs in the decades preceding the Civil War. He was active in consultations within the College about internal organization and about the revision of statutes, and in view of his increasing seniority and high reputation as a scholar, he was well qualified to represent the College in negotiations with the court, Privy Council, and legal authorities. Owing to the diplomatic efforts of Harvey and his colleagues, the integrity of the College was maintained in the face of adverse factors that were more powerful than is usually recognized in historical accounts of the College or in biographies of Harvey.

The crisis facing Harvey and his fellow members of the College of Physicians can be regarded as a necessary factor in understanding Harvey the physician, but perhaps as irrelevant or even as an inconvenient interruption of his work in the fields of physiology and embryology. However the gulf between the professional, medical, and scientific sides of Harvey's activity is not absolute. As I have demonstrated elsewhere, Harvey regarded the positive stance of his colleagues with respect to *experimental science* as fundamental for maintaining the *social status* of the academically educated physician. For the College of Physicians during the Puritan Revolution to have become identified as the uncompromising adherent of the Galenic system of medicine, would have severely added to its difficulties with the legions of its critics. Especially after 1640, following the maxims of Harvey, and utilizing his generous benefactions for the promotion of experimental science, the College successfully cultivated a modern, indeed avant-garde image.[38] But before 1640 Harvey was clearly ahead of his colleagues within the College in devoting himself to the investigation of biological problems in a manner thoroughly consistent with the "experimental philosophy" formulated by Gilbert and Bacon, and increasingly influential among Harvey's contemporaries outside the College.

Although the Fellows of the College of Physicians were not conspicuously in the vanguard of experimental philosophy, and most of them were without distinction in any field of learning, medicine in general was by no means immune to innovation. Indeed, the crisis of health, and the crisis within the medical profession described above, may be regarded as factors in a general pattern of cultural change which was highly conducive to the breakdown of traditional authoritarian values, and to diversification and innovation in medicine, science, and philosophy. Thus the most fertile phase in Harvey's scientific work, which, as indicated above, occurred before 1640, took place against the background of a distinct diversification of outlook in English medicine, and a general rise of experimental science.

An important indicator of the shifting balance within English medicine is provided by the increasing preoccupation with chemical therapy, a trend that was closely connected in intellectual circles with increasing receptivity to Paracelsian and Neoplatonic ideas. There has been a tendency to underestimate the degree to which Paracelsian medicine had already made a mark in England even before 1600. The notorious Paul Buck, whose affairs intruded into the meeting at which Harvey applied for admission as a candidate, informed the College in 1589 upon his first arraignment that his practice was largely based on Paracelsus.[39]

The cases coming to Harvey's attention during his first term as censor confirm the widespread exploitation of chemical therapy. The apothecary Edward Clark claimed to have paid £3 for medical secrets from Leonard Poe, and he was accused of administering mercury pills to one Becket.[40] The surgeons John Turner and John Collins had been administering pills containing mercury precipitate, and Turner had been prescribing mercury water at a cost of three shillings for mouth ulcers and wounds of the head. Such remedies had also been prescribed by the previously mentioned illegal practitioner and physician Thomas Lodge, a kinsman of Turner.[41] Harvey also became acquainted with the cases of James Forester and Francis Anthony, two of the most experienced and best-educated chemical practitioners.[42] Forester's revival of the chemical practice of the celebrated John Hester was boldly announced in his *Pearl of Practice* (1594). Anthony established a chemical practice in London at the turn of the century. He was accused of treating all kinds of grave diseases without license or authority. He was particularly inclined to use medicines confected from gold and mercury. When examined by the College he was found unlearned and imperfect in all facets of medicine examined. He was absolutely forbidden to practice, despite the support given his cause by three noblemen.[43] Anthony was accused of malpractice on many occasions, and mostly his delinquency involved the use of *aurum potabile*. The case brought before Harvey related to the suspicion that the death of the theologian Dr. Thomas Sanderson had been hastened by *aurum potabile*. Sanderson's treatment had cost him twenty shillings for the medicine, and forty shillings for the essence of gold.[44]

Chemical therapy was an issue at many of the meetings of the College attended by Harvey. He was present in 1611 when Jacob Domingo was accused in connection with employing mercury precipitate, arsenic, hyoscymus, and opium in the treatment of venereal disease.[45] Antimony was also frequently mentioned in cases against empirics during this period. Robert Fludd complained to his colleagues in the College that antimony cups were being freely advertised for sale at the Sign of the Magpie in Gunpowder Alley.[46] A report to the Privy Council signed by Harvey and colleagues insisted that no "grocer, apothecary, druggist or any other chemist or person may sell freely (as has generally been done) to any poor woman or the meaner sort of people [*mulierculis aut plebeculis*], arsenic, orpiment, mercury sublimate or precipitate, opium, coloquintida, scammony, hellebore, and other drugs either dangerous or poisonous." The apothecaries replied that it was pointless to place restrictions on them, since such substances were freely available from grocers and chandlers.[47]

The chemical remedy that was used by the public in perhaps the greatest quantities was *lac sulphuris*. This remedy rapidly came into prominence in England after its description in Croll's *Basilica chymica* (1609). By the 1630s, apothecaries were purchasing large quantities of sulphur and manufacturing *lac sulphuris* on an extensive scale. It was clearly a very profitable trade, which they were unwilling to relinquish. Many cases were brought against apothecaries on the grounds of retailing the drug without prescription, retailing a drug not contained in the London pharmacopoeia, for adulteration, and for manufacturing the substance in iron rather than glass containers. The *lac sulphuris* affair, more than anything else, drove the apothecaries and physicians into confrontation before the Court of Star Chamber. It was in the context of this controversy that Harvey made his plea that the apothecaries should desist from the "promiscuous" sale of drugs.[48]

Chemical therapy was perhaps championed even more by surgeons than by apothecaries. Since the late sixteenth century the antidotaries produced by English surgeons had contained a substantial representation of chemical remedies. The Paracelsian emphasis of the practice of English surgeons was confirmed in Harvey's generation in the writings of one of their leading literary spokesmen, John Woodall.[49] In 1639 an elaborate illustrated title-page was introduced into the new edition of Woodall's *Surgeon's Mate*, modelled closely on the title-page of Croll's *Basilica chymica*. Portraits of Paracelsus and other alchemical luminaries were depicted on the title-page of this important and popular handbook. This was the first time that a portrait of Paracelsus had been included in a work published in England.

Chemical therapy and the rationale provided for it by the Paracelsian medical philosophy held attractions for all grades of medical practitioner. In particular the novel, cheap, simple, and potent remedies, seemingly useful for all classes of disease, greatly increased the resources of practitioners designated as empirics by the College of Physicians. Surgeons could not be prevented from employing chemicals for internal as well as external treatments; apothecaries could easily retail simple inorganic preparations without prescription, and it was not possible to restrain others from purchasing and using indiscriminately a wide range of dangerous drugs. Thus chemical therapy was deeply subversive of the interests of the College of Physicians. However, by the time of Harvey chemical remedies were enjoying such currency that the College had little choice but to accept their selective use, and ultimately to incorporate a sizeable selection of chemical remedies into the London pharmacopoeia. Such simple and popular drugs as *lac sulphuris* were no doubt left out of the pharmacopoeia in order to limit the freedom of operation of apothecaries.

The London pharmacopoeia betokens a softening in the attitude of the College toward medical innovation. Before 1600 the Fellows had adopted an uncompromising attitude toward any critic of Galen, and they had displayed little sympathy for chemical therapy. This no doubt accounted for a strained relationship between the College and Thomas Mouffet, the leading English academic physician supporting Paracelsus. When the well-known mathematician and physician Thomas Hood was examined by the College in 1595, he frankly admitted that he had not read any of Galen's works, a surprising admission considering that he had been granted a Cambridge M.D. At his next appearance he insisted that "he had not read Galen because he could not be greatly esteemed," but he admitted acquaintance with Forester's *Pearl of Practice* and other modern writings. Not surprisingly, Hood was forbidden to practice—although shortly afterwards he was granted a license without further formalities.[50]

An interesting sign of change occurred in 1601, when the statutes were modified to remove the longstanding proscription on Fellow's engaging in alchemy or the use of quintessences.[51] Thereafter, although independently-minded alchemical physicians like Forester, Anthony, and Arthur Dee were persecuted, others, who were more compliant, were accepted as licentiates or even as fellows.[52] A test case occurred in 1605 when Robert Fludd offered himself as a candidate. Fludd had studied both at Oxford and at various continental universities in preparation for his M.D. As a noteworthy concession he was examined in both Galenic and Spagyric medicine, but was found only partly sufficient in either, with the result that he was sent away to study further, and forbidden to practice in the meantime. At his next appearance before the College, Fludd proclaimed the superiority of chemical therapy, and cried down Galenic physicians with contempt. Predictably, after this and other outbursts, Fludd's candidature was delayed, but he gradually complied with College demands. Harvey was present at his formal admission to fellowship in 1609.[53] Once admitted Fludd attended meetings more actively than Harvey, and he was just as energetic as his colleagues in opposing empirics. The immigrant French Paracelsian physician Theodore de Mayerne was positively encouraged to become a Fellow. In 1627 the College would even have amended its statutes in order to appoint him an elect.[54] Mayerne's privileged treatment is explained by his influential position as a court physician, in which capacity he was able to represent the interests of the College before the King. Mayerne played little direct part in the internal affairs of the College, but it is noticeable that he was drafted onto the committee concerned with the pharmacopoeia, and also invited to compose the Epistle Dedicatory to the King.[55] Mayerne together with Fludd, who was also involved with the pharmacopoeia, may well have exercised oversight of the section containing chemical remedies.

In contrast with their counterpart in Paris, the College of Physicians in London adopted a more accommodating position toward Paracelsian medicine. This compromise to a certain extent strengthened the position of competitors of the College, since it assisted the argument that the College was exercising an arbitrary monopoly. But this was offset by an advantage in relating the College to the increasingly influential Paracelsian and Neoplatonic movements. Metaphysical authors like John Donne set the tone of natural philosophy for Harvey's generation. Donne was not unusual in displaying a deep interest in the nature of life, the processes of disease, and the place of man in the cosmos. The complex imagery that he utilized absorbed certain elements directly from Paracelsus.[56] Robert Burton's *Anatomy of Melan-*

choly (1621) illustrates the vast range of medical authorities accessible to the Jacobean intellectual. Burton made free use of Paracelsian sources. Both Donne and Burton were laymen. In this period no rigid boundaries were drawn between scientific specialities. Many laymen participated freely in debates on medical and biological issues, just as a physician like Gilbert was not exceptional in writing on physics and cosmology. The Neoplatonic intellectual fashions of the Jacobean period almost dictated the broadest possible framework for scientific investigation, and encouraged the widest use of analogical reasoning. Robert Fludd's encyclopaedic writings, extending from mechanics to medicine, typify the catholic intellectual aspirations of Harvey's generation. Harvey's own views about the museum that he established at the College of Physicians indicate that he too regarded such a range of interests as obligatory for the learned physician.[57] It is necessary to take account of this broader context when assessing the intellectual background to Harvey's work.

In the course of stimulating departures from the scholastic framework, Neoplatonism generated fresh perspectives into the nature of vital processes, employing concepts outside the framework of Galenic physiology. Significant indications of this trend are to be found in the writings of William Gilbert, Harvey's great predecessor in the College of Physicians. Although not concerned specifically with biological questions, Gilbert carried biological insights into his studies of magnetism and cosmology. He found peripatetic categories completely inadequate to describe and explain the phenomena with which he was concerned. He departed from the norms of his fellow physicians and elaborated a cosmology that has many points of contact with that adopted by Giordano Bruno. In the opening sections of *De mundo*, Gilbert paved the way for Harvey by explicitly criticizing those who slavishly followed Aristotle and Galen, and by discarding explanations of generation and change within the universe couched in reductionist terms, with reference to atoms, or Aristotelian and Paracelsian elements. In reaction to this "impoverished" approach, Gilbert turned to the hylozoism of the ancients. He traced the origins of a more tenable viewpoint to the systems of Hermes, Zoroaster and Orpheus, which embraced the conception of a universal soul. It was essential to regard the universe as "animate, and all globes, all stars, and this glorious earth, too,...from the beginning by their own destinate souls governed, and from them also to have the impulse of self-preservation. Nor are the organs required for organic action lacking, whether implanted in the homogenic nature, or scattered through the homogenic body...."[58] Following Anaxagoras, Gilbert located the source of motion in an animistic principle that was effective in the ultimate homogenial or similar parts of matter (*homogenica pars*, or, *corporum similiarium partium*) and that acted as the seminal agencies for all vital processes (*rerum omnia semina*).[59] Against Aristotle he argued that the earth was not inert and static, but was like other planetary bodies gifted with a capacity for "circular" movement. Without such generative motion all nature would be torpid. Just as animals require incessant working of the heart and arteries, so the earth's motion was necessary for awakening its inner life.[60]

It comes as no surprise to discover Gilbert finding analogues of the organ-systems of animals throughout nature and speaking of a *circulation* of the humors between the viscera of the earth, in which the humors are carried to the surface in the veins, poured out through springs, and returned to the interior by gravitation.[61] Gilbert attached special importance to the lodestone because he supposed that it encapsulated in a microcosmic form the animistic properties of heavenly bodies or any living organism. After Thales he believed that only a soul that suffuses the whole, but also is contained in every part, could explain the capacity of a lodestone for self-movement, by which it was able to be "incited, directed, and moved in a circle."[62] No less than Giordano Bruno, Gilbert reached toward a system of correspondences by which the generation and life of all levels of existence in the universe could be explained according to uniform principles. In Gilbert's case one of the unifying factors in the animistic conception of the stars, planets, earth, and magnet was belief in their common regenerative and conservationist capacity manifest in various kinds of circular movement.

John Dee, Gilbert's older contemporary, had carried to a much greater extreme of complexity than Gilbert the elaboration of systems of geometrical, numerological, and symbolic relationships, which were posited as codes for revealing fundamental harmonies in nature. Dee and Gilbert provided sophisticated expositions of ideas that exercised great appeal in Jacobean England. While by no means representing a unified approach to the new philosophy, the two authors drew freely upon analogies between all facets of nature, each recognizing the value of quantification, and each accepting a fundamental geometrical harmony of nature.

Inevitably speculations about man played an integral part in the above systems of symbolism. These were developed at a general level by John Donne and other metaphysical writers, and at a more technical level by physicians like Robert Fludd and Sir Thomas Browne. In the present context it is noteworthy that both the idea of the primacy of the heart and of a generalized circulation played a significant part in Jacobean medical thought. John Donne dismissed the Galenic theory of the equality of brain, liver and heart in favor of the view that "the Heart alone is in the Principalitie, and in the Throne, as King, the rest as Subjects," insisting that "How little of a Man is the *Heart*, and yet it is all by which he *is*." The symbol is of life as a tension between a generative force extending from the heart toward the circumference, and a degenerative tendency from the circumference to the center.[63] Donne's writings predominantly described the cycle of human health and disease as coherent with the cycle of the seasons, and with the general hermetic symbolism relating God to the center and circumference of a circle.

The ideas just described achieved particular prominence by virtue of their relevance to the debate over the medicinal powers of *aurum potabile*. The idea that gold was a medicine for the heart was by no means new. However, *aurum potabile* seems to have attracted little attention in England before its popularization by Francis Anthony. This medicine was specifically mentioned in the first indictment of Anthony before the College of Physicians in 1600. *Aurum potabile* became central to Anthony's practice, made him universally known, and guaranteed him powerful allies in his conflicts with the College of Physicians.[64] Not only were cases relating to Anthony's use of *aurum potabile* frequently brought before the College, but the use of this medicine was at issue in a vigorous exchange of pamphlets.[65] Anthony's own writings were inspected by the College, and its representatives issued replies drawing upon a formidable list of authorities condemning the use of *aurum potabile*.

Anthony produced an erudite and convincing defence of his position. In the dedication to James I he presented the iatrochemists as the restorers of medicine from its decline under the influence of scholastic authorities. In a manner similar to Mouffet and other Paracelsians he argued for the exploitation of the medicinal properties of the rich store of minerals placed by the creator in the viscera of the earth. Anthony argued for the medicinal virtues of minerals in the context of an animistic conception of the earth very like that employed by Gilbert.[66] The second chapter of Anthony's work was devoted to validating the use of the great variety of mineral preparations that had come into daily use in medical applications. In view of the wide variety of metals of proven efficacy, he stated, it was inconsistent to deny the medicinal properties of gold, and in view of its superiority among metals, it was likely to be more medicinally efficacious than any other substance. Indeed it might become the essence of a universal medicine. Anthony argued along traditional lines that in view of the astral relationship between gold and the heart as the most noble bodies in their spheres of existence, gold would act by strengthening the heart. Thereby Anthony was led to re-emphasize the physiological dominance of the heart. The heart was the abode of life, the fount of the vital spirits and blood, bestowing on all parts movement and vitality. Natural heat and radical moisture took their existence from this single source.[67]

Anthony soon received support from an influential quarter, Michael Maier, physician to Emperor Rudolf II and later to Moritz, Landgrave of Hesse. Maier spent some time in England before 1616, completing his famous series of alchemical and emblematic works. Circumstantial evidence suggests that he was associated with Robert Fludd.[68] Maier's first work, *Arcana arcanissima*, dedicated to Sir William Paddy, a leading figure within the College of Physicians, was possibly published in London in 1614. His *Lusus serius* (Oppenheim, 1616), dealing with the imagery of mercury, was dedicated to Francis Anthony and two other chemists. *De circulo physico quadrato* (Oppenheim, 1616) was primarily an exploration of the symbolic inter-relationships between the heart, the sun, and gold. It formed a natural sequel to Anthony's *Medicinae chymicae*. An introductory poem explains the fundamentally "circular" relationship between the three prime bodies. The rays of the sun generated gold in the bowels of the earth, the sun strengthened the heart, and the heart strengthened the body, so invigorating the soul, which then served God, the source of the vital heat of the sun. By this circulation the vitality of the macrocosm and microcosm was preserved.[69] Maier described in similar terms to Anthony, the dominance of the heart as situated in the inner court (*aula*) of the body, like a prince governing all things in his state.[70] In the text Maier supported at length the view later reiterated in remarkably similar terms by Harvey, that the heart was the principal organ of the body, the first to live, last to die, and the seat of all vital processes.[71] From the heart vital heat and spirits were radiated out to the peripheries to conserve the life of the parts, and react against diseases.[72]

The writers discussed above prepared the way for the synthesis produced in the voluminous writings of Robert Fludd, who like Maier dedicated a work to Paddy.[73] Even Fludd's early unpublished work, the *Tractatus de tritico* (1619/20), represented an extension of the analogies developed by Anthony and Maier, by introducing wheat as "the only Kinge of all vegetable graines," a temple in which resides the highest vegetative virtues, its quintessence serving as a cordial equivalent in properties to the seed of gold.[74] It is now well known that Fludd went on to make extensive use of the sun-heart analogy, and various applications of the idea of circulation, in his *Anatomiae amphitheatrum* (1623), and later writings, as well as becoming the first author to make favorable reference to Harvey in a printed work, in a section of *Medicina catholica* dated 1629. In elaborating his theory of the weapon-salve Fludd, in *Anatomiae amphitheatrum* and in his above-mentioned debate with Foster, drew extensively on the ideas of Gilbert.[75]

Fludd's primary interest was in illustrating the ease with which Harveian circulation could be assimilated into the elaborate system of symbolism developed by the Neoplatonists. With varying degrees of emphasis, and with great repetitiveness in writings produced both before and after the publication of *De motu cordis,* Fludd evolved the idea that a "catholic spirit" was a fundamental expression of the *anima mundi.* The sun gave life to the planets by issuing this spirit, distributing it over the surface of the earth by circulatory air currents. The spirit found its way into the germ of wheat and the heart—tabernacles or temples that acted as microcosmic suns; the heart, by pulsating, distributed vital energies to the bodily parts by a process of circulation. Harveian circulation seemed to be a logical and appropriate pathway for this process, but Fludd's idea of circulation was by no means dependent on or always identifiable with the Harveian pathway. In man, the catholic spirit found its home in blood, which was emphatically and consistently regarded as the seat of the human soul. Blood was thought to renew its redness and virtue by means of an attractive property analogous to the power of a magnet.

The speculations of Robert Fludd exemplify the manner in which the Jacobean intellectual conceived problems of biology or medicine in a general metaphysical framework. It was not only pertinent, but almost obligatory to draw upon analogies from fields as diverse as cosmology and mechanics. It was these latter subjects which formed the center of gravity of English scientific effort at the turn of the century. It was in these areas that English experimental philosophers and mathematicians made their first major contribution to European science. Harvey was exceptional in the degree to which he concentrated on biological questions. It was common for physicians like Gilbert, Ridley, Recorde, Hood, Forster, and Bainbridge to establish their reputations as mathematicians rather than as biologists. This degree of concentration on the mathematical and physical sciences is fully consistent with the demands of the expansionist English economy in the late sixteenth century. Harvey's work occurred against a background of almost frenetic entrepreneurial and innovative activity in the fields of navigation, commerce, technology, and agriculture. Jacobean England pulsed with projects, inventors, and inventions. John Dee was deeply committed to the promotion of oceanic navigation and the extension of English fisheries; Gilbert's *De magnete* was largely concerned with navigational problems; Fludd, Mayerne and Edward Jordan utilized their skills in chemistry in schemes relating to chemical technology.[76] Typical among the scientist-projectors was Cornelius Drebbel, whose versatile activities as a hydraulic engineer, chemist, and inventor have earned him the reputation of providing the model for Bacon's Solomon's House.[77] Drebbel was primarily known by his inventions; his literary output was limited to a modest volume of essays dealing with the interconvertibility of the Aristotelian's "elements," the nature and preparation of quintessences, and finally with his famous perpetual motion, in which macrocosmic and microcosmic "circulations" were imitated by means of chemical and mechanical contrivances. Operating at a more practical and sensationalist level, Drebbel illustrated precisely the same philosophical unity and encyclopaedic range of interest in medicine, physiology, chemistry, and mechanics, as that displayed in the more erudite works of Fludd.[78]

The experiences of hydraulic engineers and inventors like Salomon de Caus and Drebbel provide the context for the speculations of Walter Warner about circulation. Walter Warner is rarely mentioned more than in passing as contributing to the emergence of circulation hypotheses in England; he is primarily remembered as the mathematician who edited the work of Thomas Harriot. Warner was firmly rooted to the Neoplatonic and alchemical tradition through his association with the circle of Ralegh and the ninth Earl of Northumberland. He published almost nothing, and most of his manuscripts were destroyed. His remaining writings, like those of his friend Harriot, deal with a wide range of topics. In a manuscript treatise on physiology almost certainly dating from before 1628, Warner expressed his belief in a universal "reciprocation or circulation," the existence of which placed the "life of animals or state of animality *in statu fluens* a state of continued flux and mutation and *in continuo fieri,* as is that of fires or flame and of the sea and the earth and indeed the whole univers."[79] Warner's "perpetual circulatory pneumato-hydraulic motion" involved the regular suction of blood from the veins to the heart and its consequent dispersal from the heart to the arteries.[80] By this means the animal spirit was continually replenished in the organs of the body. Warner was so unspecific about the structure of the cardio-vascular system that it is not clear whether his circulatory device differed more than marginally from that adopted by Fludd.

However as Warner's terminology suggests, he was much less committed to geometrical analogies than Dee, and much more concerned than Fludd with mechanical models, in framing his circulatory system. In applying hydraulic principles Warner was brought to many of the same conclusions as

Harvey with respect to the motion of the heart. It was firmly decided that the blood could not be the direct cause of its own motion. The heart was responsible for circulation, being suited for this purpose by its muscular structure which brought about a regular "voluntary dilatation and contraction." Warner noted that an excised heart continued to pulsate. The contraction of the fibres of the heart was responsible for the expulsion of blood into the arteries at systole, and the extraction or exsuction of blood from the veins in diastole.[81] The arteries themselves played no active part in the pulse, acting merely as "dead pipes" through which the blood was driven.[82] Although weak on matters of anatomical detail, and silent on certain crucial issues, Warner's discussion of circulation has a sufficient number of points of identity with the work of Harvey, for it to cause no surprise that a widespread rumor developed among their contemporaries that Harvey had at least obtained the hint of his discovery from the elderly mathematician.[83]

It has not been the purpose of the present paper to rake over dead coals on the question of Harvey's precursors. No amount of investigation of background and context has reduced the stature of Harvey's *De motu cordis*. Nevertheless it is clear that the social and intellectual climate of Jacobean England is relevant to our full understanding of the preoccupations of Harvey the physician, and for at least explaining the receptivity of his countrymen to the theory of circulation.

In Harvey's own work, one is impressed by the singularity of many of his interests. His initiative in exploiting comparative anatomy and vivisection clearly owed little to his contemporaries in England. The immediate context for his work on the cardiovascular system and embryology was provided by the investigations of anatomists in the Italian tradition. These factors were fundamental for establishing the definitive status of the Harveian theory of circulation. The positive role played in Harvey's work by the emergent experimental philosophy and by the vigorous school of mathematical practitioners in England is difficult to assess. Harvey was clearly aware of work in such fields as magnetism and hydraulics. His family and social situation of necessity familiarized him with the broader commercial and economic context.[84] He used mechanical analogies freely and sensitively, avoiding many of the crudities of Cartesian mechanistic physiology. His use of the analogy of the heart to the water-bellows and later to the fire-engine (*sipho*) was particularly important and perceptive.[85] Harvey's conception of the cardiovascular structure as a hydraulic system, in both terminological detail and general framework, owed something to the work of the hydraulic engineers who were so active at the period in devising structures involving the use of valves and water under pressure, from architectural waterworks to mine drainage pumps. These experiences may have assisted Harvey (like Leonardo a century before) to think more realistically than other anatomists about the dynamics of the circulatory system.

The affinity between Harvey and his Neoplatonic contemporaries becomes ever closer at the points where he moves from the descriptive to the explanatory level in questions relating to both circulation and generation. The relevance of pre-Harveian circulatory hypotheses to the formulation of the Harveian mechanism of circulation must remain an unanswered question. Perhaps this possibility is given somewhat greater credence the greater the length of the time-lag in composition posited between the *Praelectiones* and first section of the *De motu cordis* on the one hand, and the second, circulatory section of *De motu cordis* on the other.[86]

It is clear that Harvey was not merely concerned with conducting his work at the level of case studies in experimental biology which could be resolved definitely in terms of the techniques and indubitable scientific knowledge available at his period. His work on physiology reached toward the solution of the problem of the nature of life, and his embryological studies related to his search into the nature of final causes. These two poles of his work can be regarded as complementary aspects of a unified biological philosophy.[87] Inevitably these problems carried Harvey into the realms of metaphysical speculation in which he showed himself familiar with the currents of thought expressed in the literature discussed above. His approach to problems was characteristically single-minded, and he avoided the more unsophisticated models of the hermeticists. Nevertheless, in discussing the physiological role of the heart and blood, or the nature of generation, his Aristotelianism became infused with ideas derived from Biblical and Neoplatonic sources. As in the case of Gilbert's speculations about magnetism, reductionist explanations based on atoms or Aristotelian and Paracelsian elements were discarded as being too limited. Like Gilbert, Harvey turned to hylozoic theories derived from pre-Socratic sources. The magnet and the heart respectively were identified as encapsulating the properties of the similar or homogenic parts, the sources of the life of the earth, and the life of man. The lodestone and blood were animate, infused with an *anima*, as a dimension of the *anima mundi*. They thereby partook of the element of the stars. By this device the microcosm of man and the microcosm of the earth were harmoniously linked with the macrocosm of the heavens in a single comprehensive explanation.[88]

The deepening crisis of health, the assault on the authority of the College of Physicians, and the open competition between proponents of rival medical philosophies, were important factors tending to enrich the medical culture of Jacobean England. Many of the medical developments in this period, such as the controversies involving Anthony and Fludd, Primerose's critique of Harvey, the rise of chemotherapy, the *lac sulphuris* dispute, or the appearance of the *Pharmacopoeia Londinensis,* can only be understood with reference to intraprofessional conflict, and its general social context. Figures like Anthony, Maier, and Fludd may seem obscure to the modern reader, but they as much as the metaphysical poets were seen by contemporaries as representative of flourishing and progressive intellectual movements. Circumstances were prejudicial to the maintenance of the authority of Galenism, and conducive to innovation both at the philosophical and therapeutic level. It is therefore entirely to be expected that the Jacobean period should have been marked by an epidemic Paracelsianism, and by the emergence of a philosophical outlook which had many points of contact with the biological philosophy of William Harvey. It was therefore not necessary for Harvey to have access to relatively inaccessible writings by figures like Giordano Bruno, to obtain defenses of the primacy of the heart, elaborations of the vitalistic role of the blood, biological applications of the principle of circulation, examples of the use of hydraulic analogies for the cardiovascular system, or a dynamic conception of biological processes. These beliefs were by 1628 common currency in the medical culture of his age. Thus Harvey's work is undoubtedly inspired, distinctive and original, but it may also be regarded as a consistent expression of the epistemological shift occasioned by the culture of the Baroque period.[89]

Notes

1. E. A. Wrigley, "A Simple Model of London's Importance in Changing English Society and Economy 1650-1750," in P. Abrams and E. A. Wrigley, *Towns in Societies: Essays in Economic History and Historical Sociology* (Cambridge: University Press, 1978), pp. 215-43; F. P. Wilson, *The Plague in Shakespeare's London* (Oxford: Clarendon, 1927), pp. 208-15. The following general sources will be referred to specifically only when relevant for expanding a particular point in the text: Sir G. N. Clark, *A History of the Royal College of Physicians,* vol. 1 (Oxford: Clarendon, 1964); G. L. Keynes *The Life of William Harvey* (Oxford: Clarendon, 1966); C. Wall, H. C. Cameron and E. A. Underwood, *A History of the Worshipful Society of Apothecaries of London,* vol. 1 (London: Oxford Univ. Press, 1963); W. Munk, *The Roll of the Royal College of Physicians of London,* 2nd ed., 3 vols. (London, 1878).
2. C. Creighton, *A History of Epidemics in Britain,* 2nd ed., 2 vols. (London: Cass, 1965), vol. 1, pp. 475-8, 511; J. F. D. Shrewsbury, *A History of Bubonic Plague in the British Isles* (Cambridge: University Press, 1971), pp. 267-8, 333-4. See also *The Plague Reconsidered. A New Look at Its Origins and Effects in 16th and 17th Century England.* Local Population Studies Supplement (Cambridge, 1977).
3. N. McClure (ed.), *The Letters of John Chamberlain,* 2 vols. (Philadelphia: American Philosophical Society, 1939), vol. 2, pp. 576, 578-79, letters of August and September 1624. Chamberlain noted that "mortalitie is spred far and neere; and takes hold of whole housholds in many places." Detailed mortality statistics are included in letters of Joseph Mede to Sir Martin Stuteville (Wilson, *Plague in Shakespeare's London,* pp. 146, 161), and in Thomas Dekker: *The Blacke Rod* (London, 1630).

4. Thomas Dekker, *The Magnificent Entertainment* (1604), in *Dramatic Works*, ed. R. H. Shepherd (1873), i, 277. *A Rod for Run-aways* (1603), in F. P. Wilson (ed.), *The Plague Tracts of Thomas Dekker* (Oxford: Clarendon, 1925), pp. 138–39.

5. Dekker, *A Rod for Run-aways*, in Wilson, *Plague Tracts*, pp. 150–51. See also Wilson, *Plague in Shakespeare's London*. London, Royal College of Physicians, MS Annals hereafter Annals, 1 December 1625. The Annals of the College are quoted with the kind permission of the President and Fellows.

6. Donne, "An Anatomy of the World: The First Anniversary," II. 91–94, 159–60.

7. C. M. Cipolla, *Public Health and the Medical Profession in the Renaissance* (Cambridge: Univ. Press, 1976), pp. 11–66.

8. C. Webster, "Thomas Linacre and the Foundation of the College of Physicians," in F. Maddison, M. Pelling and C. Webster (eds.), *Linacre Studies*, I, (Oxford, 1977), pp. 198–222.

9. Sir William Paddy, John Argent, and Simeon Fox: Annals, 21 April 1625. Wilson, *Plague in Shakespeare's London*, p. 21.

10. Annals, 15 March 1630. *Acts of the Privy Council May 1629–May 1630* (London, 1960), Nos. 992, 1000, 18 March 1630. Keynes, *Harvey*, pp. 190–91.

11. Perhaps John Anthony, MD, son of Francis Anthony; and Jacob Domingo. Wilson, *Plague in Shakespeare's London*, p. 21. Thomas Lodge had published his *Treatise of the Plague* (London, 1603), specifically for the benefit of the poor, and in the hope of recommending his services to the civic authorities.

12. Thomas Dekker, *The Wonderfull Yeare* (1603), in *Plague Tracts*, p. 36.

13. Dekker, *Wonderful Year*, pp. 33, 37. It was commented of Thorius that when the plague raged in London, "he acted more for the public (by exposing his person too much) than his own dear concern": A. Wood, *Athenae Oxonienses*, ed. Bliss, (Oxford, 1813–20), i, 422.

14. Annals, 3 February 1625/26. Two leading apothecaries quoted Magna Carta in favor of their right to display and sell any wares: London, Guildhall Library, Apothecaries' Society, Star Chamber 1634–35, MS. 8286 fol. 2.

15. Milton, *Areopagitica* (1644), in *Complete Prose Works*, vol. II, ed. D. Sirluck (New Haven: Yale University Press, 1959), p. 535.

16. Annals, 4 May 1603. Keynes, *Harvey*, pp. 39–40. At the same meeting the Fellows faced a confrontation with Paul Buck, one of the most persistent delinquents active at this period.

17. Annals, 5 October 1604; 16 May, 5 June 1607.

18. For Elwyn, See Munk, *Roll*, i, 122. Harvey's father-in-law and Fellow of the College Lancelot Browne in 1605 attempted unsuccessfully to secure Harvey's appointment as successor to Elwyn as physician to the Tower of London: Keynes, *Harvey*, pp. 44–5. Other cases treated favorably compared with Harvey were Matthew Gwynne, Thomas Rawlins, Thomas Hearne and Matthew Lister.

19. Annals, 3, 9, 10 December 1629. 9 January, 15 March 1629/30. G. Whitteridge, *William Harvey and the Circulation of the Blood* (London: Elsevier, 1971), pp. 255–56. Primerose, *Exercitationes in librum De motu cordis adversus G. Harveum* (London, 1630).

20. Annals, 11 May 1604.

21. Annals, 18 April 1614.

22. Annals, 3 December 1613; 14 January, 4 February 1613/14.

23. Francis Anthony, M.A. 1574, M.D. 1608: Annals, 18 April 1614. First appearance before the College: Annals, 5 July 1600. James Forester, M.A. 1583: Annals, 23 August 1614. First appearance: Annals, 7 December 1592. Nicholas Fiske, undergraduate of Benet Hall, Cambridge: Annals, 4 March 1613/14.

24. Annals, 29 November 1613, 4 February 1613/14. First appearance: Annals, 7 February 1605/06.

25. Annals, 3, 15 December 1613.

26. Annals, 24 January, 21 February 1616/17. Clark, *History of the College of Physicians*, i, 235–38; J. Donnison, *Midwives and Medical Men* (London: Heinemann, 1977), pp. 13–15. J. H. Aveling, *English Midwives* (London, 1872), pp. 22–46.

27. Annals, 23 May 1614. A group of apothecaries first petitioned for separation in the spring of 1614.

28. Annals, 14 February 1614/15: "inter apothecarios errata corrigantur, idque propositum, ab aromatariis separentur, sic fore veros probos."

29. Annals, 25 June 1614: "De dispensatorio communi in officinis pharmacopoeorum habendo proponitur e Bergomensi, Norembergensi et caeteris antidotariis."

30. Annals, Michaelmas 1617, 20 February, 20 March 1617/18, 25 September 1618.

31. For further details see Wall, Cameron and Underwood, *Society of Apothecaries,* pp. 8-22, 216-20; G. Urdang (ed.), *Pharmacopoeia Londinensis of 1618. Reproduced in Facsimile with a Historical Introduction by George Urdang* (Madison: State Historical Society of Wisconsin, 1944).

32. Annals, June-December 1624.

33. Annals, 30 May, 25 June 1632.

34. Annals, 4 July 1632. Keynes, *Harvey,* pp. 81-82.

35. William Foster, *Hoplocrismi-spongus: or, a sponge to wipe away the weapon-salve* (London, 1631); Fludd, *Answer unto M. Foster* (London, 1631), pp. 122-23. Foster was son of William Foster, barber-surgeon.

36. Annals, 4 July 1634.

37. Guildhall Library, Society of Apothecaries, Star Chamber 1634-35, MS. 8286, fol. 14.

38. C. Webster, *The Great Instauration: Science, Medicine and Reform 1626-1660* (London: Duckworth, 1975), pp. 315-23.

39. See my forthcoming study, "Alchemical and Paracelsian Medicine," in Webster (ed.), *Health, Medicine and Mortality in the Sixteenth Century* (CUP). Annals, 6 June 1589.

40. Annals, 13 October 1613.

41. Annals, 13 December 1613.

42. Annals, 18 April, 23 August 1614.

43. Annals, 5 July, 7 November 1600.

44. Annals, 16 April 1614.

45. Annals, 19 January 1610/11.

46. Annals, 3 April 1637. Other cases of poisoning by antimony were reported by various members, including Harvey. A woman practitioner was accused of administering antimony. Annals, 3 August 1627. The fervent exponent of the use of antimony John Evans, author of *The Universal Medicine* (London, 1634), sold his medicine from Gunpowder Alley, Fetter Lane.

47. Annals, 30 May 1632. Guildhall Library, Society of Apothecaries, Record Book 1621-40, MS. 8205, fols. 10-12. Wall, Cameron and Underwood, *Society of Apothecaries,* pp. 45-6, 261-3.

48. Guildhall, MS. 8286. Wall, Cameron and Underwood, *Society of Apothecaries,* pp. 48-57, 266-96. Annals, 4 July 1634.

49. Webster, "Alchemical and Paracelsian medicine"; A. G. Debus, "John Woodall, Paracelsian surgeon," *Ambix,* 1962, *10:* 71-97.

50. Annals, 17 October 1595; 25 February, 5 April 1597.

51. Clark, *College of Physicians,* i, 96, 179, 384: "Nemo collega exercebit omnino alchymiam nec in curationibus utetur quinta quam vocant essentia."

52. Arthur Dee, son of John Dee, first appeared before the College in 1606: Annals, 4 April 1606.

53. Annals, 8 November 1605; 2 May 1606: "medicamentis suis chymicis praedicasse, medicos autem Galenicos cum contemptu deicisse"; Annals, 20 September 1609.

54. Annals, 5 July 1616, 27 November 1627.

55. Annals, 20 March 1617/18.

56. D. C. Allen, "John Donne's knowledge of Renaissance medicine," *English and Germanic Philology,* 1943, *42:* 322-42.

57. Keynes, *Harvey,* p. 402.

58. Gilbert, *De magnete* (1600), trans. P. F. Mottelay (London, 1893), p. 309.

59. Gilbert, *De mundo nostro sublunari philosophia nova* (Amsterdam, 1651), p. 41 & *passim*. The posthumously published *De mundo* was composed at about the same time as *De magnete*. It was widely circulated in manuscript form after Gilbert's death.

60. Gilbert, *De magnete*, p. 338.

61. Gilbert, *De mundo*, p. 291: "Terrestrem globum unum corpus, terrarum & aquarum mutuis cohaerentiis & consensu esse connexum, defluere in terra humorem suis scaturiginibus naturaliter sursum, deorsum, circulariter inter viscera, effluere referatis venis, defluere suis ponderibus, perinde ac longissimis fluminibus, vel in aperto circulariter moveri."

62. *De magnete*, p. 109.

63. John Donne, *Devotions upon Emergent Occasions*, ed. A. Raspa (Montreal/London: McGill-Queen's University Press, 1975), pp. 56-57.

64. For probable early references to Anthony's practice, see Thomas Dekker, *The Wonderful Year*, p. 37; Ben Jonson, *Volpone* (1605), I, iv, 72-74:"This is true physic, this is your sacred medicine/No talk of opiates to this great elixir/...'Tis *aurum palpibile*, if not *potabile*."

65. Francis Anthony, *Medicinae chymicae et veri potabilis auri assertio* (Cambridge, 1610); idem, *The apologie concerning a medicine called aurum potabile* (London, 1616); idem, *Panacea aurea sive tractatus duo de ipsius auro potabile* (Hamburg, 1618). Anthony's critics included: Matthew Gwynne, *Aurum non aurum* (London, 1611); Thomas Rawlins, *Admonitio de pseudochymicis* (London, 1611); John Cotta, *Cotta contra Antonium* (Oxford, 1623). The fullest account of Anthony is contained in A. Kippis (ed.), *Biographia Britannica*, 2nd ed., vol. 1 (London, 1778), pp. 221-25. For Baldwin Hamey's private remonstration with Anthony in 1610, see J. J. Keevil, *Hamey the Stranger* (London: G. Bles, 1952), pp. 113-15.

66. Anthony, *Medicinae chymicae*, pp. 25-27.

67. Anthony, *Medicinae chymicae*, pp. 27-28: "Cordi videlicet, quod domicilium est vitae, Cor scaturigo est vitalis spiritus & sanguis, omnibus reliquis membris motum & vigorem impertiens. Hic vigent nativus ille calor & humidum primogenium foventum vitae & ex hac solo forte illa primo derivantur."

68. F. Yates, *The Rosicrucian Enlightenment* (London/Boston: Routledge & Kegan Paul, 1972), pp. 80-82.

69. Maier, *De circulo physico*, p. 7:"Utque Deus Soli, Sol auro, hoc denique cordi/Vim dat, & hoc verso respicit orbe Deum:/Omnia ab hoc & ad hunc mortalia condita tendunt,/Circulus hic, quia quid constat ubique, replet." In *Atalanta fugiens* (Oppenheim, 1617), Emblem XXI, Maier discussed generation in terms of circle symbolism.

70. Maier, *De circulo physico*, p. 6.

71. Maier, *De circulo physico*, pp. 69-70: "Adhaec si cor est focus caloris, si centrum corporis humani, non Geometricè, sed Physicè intelligendo, si Rex & Princeps membrorum omnium, quo salvo caetera salva, laeso laesa sunt, si primum vivens & ultimum moriens in animali, si est sedis affectuum gravissimorum, irae, laetitiae & similium...."

72. Maier, *De circulo physico*, p. 70.

73. Fludd, *Medicina Catholica* (Frankfurt a.M., 1629-31).

74. C. H. Josten, "Robert Fludd's 'Philosophical Key' and his alchemical experiment on wheat," *Ambix*, 1963, *11*: 1-23; p. 16. Fludd's *Tractatus de tritico* was referred to before its publication in Maier's *Atalanta Fugiens*, p. 35, and later made the introductory section of *Anatomiae Amphitheatrum* (1623). For the concept of the "primacy" of wheat, see *ibid.*, pp. 11-12.

75. A. G. Debus, "Robert Fludd and the circulation of the blood," *J. Hist. Med.*, 1961, *16*: 374-93; idem, "Robert Fludd and the use of Gilbert's *De magnete* in the weapon-salve controversy," *J. Hist. Med.*, 1964, *19*: 389-417.

76. Webster, *The Great Instauration*, pp. 324-54; J. Thirsk, *Economic Policy and Projects. The Development of a Consumer Society in Early Modern England* (Oxford: University Press, 1978).

77. R. L. Colie, "Cornelius Drebbel and Salomon de Caus: Two Jacobean models for Salomon's House," *Huntington Library Quarterly,* 1954/55, *18:* 245-60.

78. Cornelius Drebbel, *Tractatus duo: prior de natura elementorum...posterior de quinta essentia...Epistola de perpetui mobilis inventione* (Hamburg, 1621). Drebbel described his invention as being "vivis instrumentis." It was probably first described in a prefatory letter to Johann Ernst Burggrave, *Biolychnium seu lucerna* (Leyden, 1610), p. 51. This latter work is relevant to the present study in view of its emphasis on the primacy of blood and on a consideration of the cosmic influences effecting the regeneration of the vital properties of blood. Burggrave's book attracted much attention among mid-century English physiologists. Drebbel's perpetual motion was first described and illustrated in a work printed in England by the Paracelsian author Thomas Twyne, *A Dialogue Philosophicall* (London, 1612), pp. 60-63.

79. British Library, MS. Birch 4934, fol. 161v. H. P. Bayon dates this manuscript c. 1610: *Proc. Roy. Soc. Med. Section Hist. Med.,* 1938/39, *32:* 711. Walter Warner (c. 1560-1643) was employed in the household of the alchemist Henry Percy, ninth Earl of Northumberland, and was primarily in charge of his library. Warner's few surviving papers are mainly located in MS. Birch 4934-4936.

80. MS. Birch 4934, fol. 139r.

81. MS. Birch 4934, fols. 137v-138r.

82. MS. Birch 4934, fols. 174r-v.

83. Warner's ideas about the circulation of blood were noted by a variety of commentators, including Aubrey, Wood and Boyle, as well as an anonymous writer in Bodleian Library, MS. Rawlinson B 158, fols. 152-53. See H. P. Bayon, "Allusions to the 'Circulation' of the Blood in MSS. anterior to *De motu cordis* 1628," *Proc. Roy. Soc. Med. Section Hist. Med.,* 1938/39, *32:* 707-18.

84. Harvey's five younger brothers were involved in trade, being connected with the Grocers', Levant, and East India companies. There are certain suggestive analogies between dynamic conceptions that emerged in the two fields of economics and physiology at the time of Harvey's work on circulation. The period 1620-1623 was marked by a particularly fertile economic debate in England. Among the contributions on the balance of trade question was Edward Misselden's *The Circle of Commerce* (London, 1623). Misselden believed that with respect to the balance of trade "all rivers of Trade spring out of this source and empty themselves again into this Ocean. All the waight of Trade falles to this center, & comes within the circuit of this Circle" (p. 142). Lewis Roberts dedicated his *Merchants Map of Commerce* (London, 1638) to William Harvey and his brothers. See B. E. Supple, *Commercial Crisis and Change in England 1600-1642* (Cambridge: At the University Press, 1959).

85. C. Webster, "William Harvey's Conception of the Heart as a Pump," *Bull. Hist. Med.,* 1965, *39:* 508-17.

86. J. J. Bylebyl, "The Growth of Harvey's *De motu cordis,"* *Bull. Hist. Med.,* 1973, *47:* 427-70.

87. For a detailed examination of this subject see W. Pagel, *William Harvey's Biological Ideas* (Basel/New York: Phiebig, 1967); *New Light on William Harvey* (Basel/New York: S. Karger, 1975).

88. See especially *De motu cordis,* chapter 8; *De generatione,* Ex. 71, 72. For Harvey's critique of Aristotle, Paracelsus, and the atomists, and for his theory of similar or homogeneous parts above the status of the elements, see *De generatione* (London, 1651), pp. 486-88.

89. Although drawing upon rather different sources of evidence, this conclusion is broadly in line with H. Sigerist, "William Harvey's Stellung in der europäischen Geistesgeschichte," *Archiv für Kulturgeschichte,* 1928, *19:* 158-68, and W. Pagel, "The Position of Harvey and Van Helmont in the History of European Thought," *J. Hist. Med.,* 1958, *13:* 186-99.

The Medical Side of Harvey's Discovery: The Normal and the Abnormal

Jerome J. Bylebyl

By the medical side of Harvey's discovery, I mean the various ways in which his recognition of the circulation was affected by the fact that he was a physician, concerned with the cause and treatment of disease, as well as with the functions of the body in a state of health. As a dietetic physician, Harvey had been trained to regard all bodily functions as subject to great variation in response to a wide range of factors, both physical and psychological, and further to see such changes as potential causes of disease. He had also been taught to look upon the various aspects of therapy as so many ways of manipulating this functional variability in order to avert or cure disease. Such considerations were of particular importance with regard to the movement of the blood, because no other function was thought to be more highly susceptible to dramatic change in response to circumstances, and few were more frequently the object of direct therapeutic manipulation. As a result, the pre-Harveian conceptions of the normal movement of the blood were highly immune to direct empirical refutation, because any given phenomenon that was inconsistent with these ideas would routinely be interpreted as the abnormal result of the particular conditions under which it occurred. In fact, all the elements of the circulation were reasonably familiar to Harvey's predecessors, but some of them were specifically regarded as unusual, if not downright dangerous, patterns of blood flow.

Accordingly, a crucial factor in Harvey's discovery was the subtle process of redefining the distinction between what is normal and what is abnormal, between what is special effect and what is constant process. As we shall see, Harvey was for many years inclined to draw this line in much the same way as his predecessors had done, so that for him as for them the circulation remained hidden under a series of presumed special effects. But on the other hand, as the theory of circulation eventually took shape in his mind, it was indeed a startling new physiological principle, but one which owed a great deal to older pathological and therapeutic notions.

Dietetics and Physiology[1]

As mentioned, the basic conditions for the discovery were set by the ancient Greek conception of dietetic medicine, which accorded a place of central importance to physiological knowledge,[2] but which also placed heavy demands and limitations upon such knowledge. To illustrate the situation, we may refer to a traditional formulation according to which the factors influencing health and disease were divided into the natural, the non-natural, and the contra-natural.[3] The things natural are the inherent constituents, faculties, and activities of the healthy organism. The science of these things was called "physiology," and corresponded approximately to what is still meant by that term.[4] From the medical point of view, the things natural provided a basic set of factors which are essential to life, but which are subject to great variation to produce either a healthy or a diseased state of life.

The non-naturals, by contrast, are those things which are able to cause such variation in the natural constituents and functions.[5] The traditional list usually included the ambient air, exercise and rest, sleep and waking, things taken in, things excreted and retained, and passions of the soul (i.e., strong emotions). These are also essential aspects of life, but the individual has more or less control over the particular ways in which they are used—e.g., how much and what kind of food he eats—and they can be either helpful, harmful, or indifferent, depending upon how he exercises these options.

Most changes in the internal functions resulting from the non-naturals will be only transient variations of one kind or another, but if carried beyond a certain point they can have more long-lasting effects in the form of disease.[6] This brings us to the things contrary to nature, which include diseases, their causes, and their symptoms.[7] The disease is essentially a *functio laesa,* i.e., one of the patient's inherent bodily processes in a state of disorder. The cause will encompass both the extrinsic factors which brought about this situation, and some resulting internal factor, such as an excess of a humor, which is the immediate cause of the functional disruption. The symptoms, in turn, are the externally manifest consequences of the disordered function. However, traditional medicine also attached great importance to the inherent power of the body to heal itself, so that some of the functional alterations will represent such efforts to overcome the internal cause of the disease and restore health.[8]

The role of the physician, then, is to have a thorough knowledge of the natural bodily functions, and how and why they can be changed to result in disease. He must also have an intimate knowledge of the variations in the manifest signs and symptoms associated with these processes, in order to be able to judge the patient's state of health or disease, and, in the event of disease, to be able to predict the outcome of the natural healing process. On this basis he will then provide the patient with detailed advice on how to regulate his use of the non-naturals, in order to preserve health if he is healthy, to restore health if he is not, or to assist the body's healing efforts if he is actually sick. In addition, the physician might prescribe more active forms of therapeutic intervention, which would usually be intended to reinforce the natural healing process, but which would not be necessary if the body were able to achieve the same result spontaneously. Thus, the physician would also regard his own ministrations as an active determinant of the patient's internal bodily processes, and for obvious psychological reasons he would tend to think that he had more rather than less power in this regard.

As one might expect, the body of physiological theory which evolved within such a medical context was heavily influenced by it. For one thing, traditional physiology portrayed the organism as a relatively unstable entity, susceptible to great variation in response to all manner of circumstance.[9] The physiological—the inherent constituents and functions of the body—provided the substrate for this change, but any bodily phenomenon not directly related to the manifest, persisting activities of the healthy organism would be regarded as the transient result of particular circumstances. Even such common events as sleep and emotions were consistently looked upon as affections of the truly permanent bodily functions, rather than being seen as functions in their own right.

Furthermore, not only did physiological theory need to allow for manifold variability in the organism, but to be of value to a physician it also had to be able to account for the known consequences of disease and the effects of therapeutic intervention.[10] Accordingly, physicians tended to define their conceptions of normal function not only with reference to the activities of the healthy organism, but also in relation to their professional experience of disease and therapy, which provided both positive insights as well as negative points of contrast for understanding the state of health.[11] However, simply to state the alternatives of either a positive or a negative relationship is to suggest the potential pitfalls in a conception of the normal that is too heavily derived from experience of the abnormal. In extreme form it could lead to a view of the normal as little more than the absence of various overtly pathological conditions. And even supposing that a process such as inflammation has some positive physiological analogue, there are any number of ways in which the latter might be conceived. It might, for example, be a more moderate form of the disease process, but it might equally be its diametric opposite.[12]

Moreover, in some cases it was not just a matter of drawing on the experience of disease to define the normal order of things, but of expanding an existing pathological theory into a new physiological corollary. This was especially likely to occur because in the early formative period of Greek medical theory, as represented by many of the treatises in the Hippocratic corpus, the chief interest lay in the processes of disease and healing.[13] Out of this emerged some fundamental theoretical concepts which subsequently exerted a major influence not only on pathological theories, but on efforts to define and explain the functions of health as well.[14]

Physicians played a major role in the development of these later, more comprehensive physiological theories, but the initial impetus toward their formation seems to have come from the ancient natural philosophers, who were understandably more concerned with the healthy organism than with problems of disease and therapy.[15] Moreover, one of the philosophers, namely Aristotle, introduced the method of systematic animal dissection on a broadly comparative basis, and this, in conjunction with a teleological point of view, provided a greatly expanded perspective on the internal workings of the body. Before long these concerns and methods were taken up by physician-scientists, who extended them to include human dissection, as well as some vivisection, both animal and (by some accounts) human. These investigations produced some very important results, such as the discovery of both the existence and the functions of the nervous system. And these findings in turn provided new insights into disease processes, in addition to having significant therapeutic implications.[16]

Biological research thus had a quite palpable influence on medical thought and practice, but it did not change the fundamental relationship between physiological theory and dietetic medicine, as described above. For one thing, the number of ancient physicians who actually engaged in such research was not very large, and a sizeable segment of the medical profession was actively hostile to these pursuits, maintaining that accumulated experience was the only reliable basis for the practice of medicine.[17] Furthermore, the relatively few ancient physician-scientists were themselves more or less busily engaged in the practice of medicine, so that their deliberate researches tended to interact with, rather than supercede, their experience of disease and therapy in shaping their outlook on physiological questions. And, along with experience and research, the authority of the Hippocratic corpus carried great weight for many ancient physicians, and this ensured that traditional pathological theories would continue to exert a major influence on the development of physiological thought. Galen, in particular, was second to none in his dedication to anatomical and physiological research, but he was quite convinced that one of the major results of such studies would be to confirm and elucidate the medical doctrines of Hippocrates.[18]

Moreover, the concerns and needs of the dietetic physician not only worked their influence at the theoretical level, they could even rebound upon the very methods of biological investigation. Almost from the earliest days of anatomical research we find the argument that a given observation is misleading or inconclusive because it represents a post-mortem change in the body, not a true reflection of the normal situation. This was not strictly a physician's argument, since it was used by Aristotle himself on occasion, but it accorded well with the dietetic presumption that the body is indeed readily susceptible to such change.[19] In fact, for those ancient physicians who opposed anatomical research it served as a comprehensive indictment of the whole method.[20]

It was possibly in response to this charge of post-mortem change that the practice of vivisection was first introduced by the ancient medical anatomists, but if anything the problems here were even worse.[21] For cutting into the bodies of living creatures could not be sharply distinguished from such overtly violent situations as deliberate or accidental trauma, the execution of criminals, animal sacrifice, or simple butchery. The closest analogue, namely surgery, had more salutary connotations, but even so, the good surgeon was acutely aware that he could do great harm by a slip of the knife. Furthermore, in the absence of anaesthesia the subjects of such experiments would be undergoing violent struggles and extreme emotions, both of which could, on dietetic theory, profoundly change their internal functions. Thus there were always ample grounds for challenging a vivisectional demonstration as an unnatural result of the method itself.[22] And even more insidiously, the vivisector himself would approach the operation prepared to encounter such distortions. In fact, until well into modern times the basic aim of most vivisectional procedures was to elucidate some normal function not by making it more manifest, but precisely by destroying it.[23]

These circumstances were still much the same for Harvey as they had been for his ancient predecessors. He did, of course, accord an important place to observations and experiments in live animals, but a glance at *De motu cordis* will show that the results of such studies were freely intermingled not only with the findings of comparative, human, and pathological anatomy, but also with experience of disease and trauma, and the effects of therapeutic procedures, in human patients.[24] All of these contributed significantly to his physiological theories, and he clearly expected such theories in turn to shed important light on pathological and therapeutic issues. Furthermore, Harvey never gave up the basic assumption of dietetic medicine, that the internal bodily functions are subject to dramatic change in response to circumstances. Accordingly, he was acutely aware of the possibility that a given vivisectional observation might represent a gross distortion of the normal function, and therefore went to considerable lengths to reassure both himself and his readers that he had not been misled in this way.[25] Indeed, he was himself prepared to argue that an opposing view may have been mistakenly derived from the observation of post-mortem changes, and even to suggest that the result of an experiment described by Galen was rendered problematic by the reaction of "the living body."[26]

Moreover, Harvey directed his attention to an aspect of bodily function where all of these problems of indeterminacy were present in the most extreme degree. For in the views of his predecessors and contemporaries there was almost no extrinsic circumstance which could not have a more or less dramatic effect on the movement of the blood, in rate as well as direction. This attitude was due in part to the fact that such movements or their effects do not actually become manifest except under unusual circumstances. But the association of abnormality with the movement of the blood was greatly reinforced by the close link between dietetic medicine and humoral theory, which looked to changes in the quality, quantity, and distribution of the bodily fluids, above all the blood, as the most important internal consequences of the use or misuse of the non-naturals. Furthermore, much of traditional therapy was aimed at inducing the blood to undergo patterns of movement which it would not do otherwise, so that any investigative technique one might employ to study the movement of the blood could also be presumed to be the cause of any movement which it revealed.

The obstacles to any reliable conclusions about the movement of the blood would thus seem to have been insurmountable, and yet Harvey obviously overcame them. However, he did so not because he immediately saw through these pervasive presuppositions, but because he originally set out to study quite another function, namely the movement of the heart, which was relatively free from such problems of uncertainty. For the heartbeat is the one internal bodily function whose steady occurrence throughout life is perhaps most readily apparent, and it had also proven quite amenable to direct observation. There are descriptions in Homer of battle wounds involving the beating heart,[27] and in an anonymous treatise on the heart dating from the third century B.C. it is reported that one can "observe the heart tossing about as a whole, but the auricles independently inflating and collapsing."[28] Galen gave detailed directions for exposing the beating heart of a live animal, and in contrast to many of his other vivisections which were aimed at selectively destroying some function, here the whole emphasis was on preserving normal conditions in order to make the heartbeat available for positive scrutiny.[29] He particularly stressed the importance of not collapsing the lungs, and Vesalius later picked up on this point to develop the method of artificial insufflation in order to make the living heart even more accessible.[30] And Harvey continued this methodological thrust in a different way by using cold blooded animals—as he put it, "if someone dissects a living snake, he will see its heart beat distinctly and placidly for more than an hour."[31] Thus it was no coincidence that the reform of physiological thought should have stemmed from the study of this particular phenomenon, which can be directly observed to occur in such a seemingly normal way.

This is not to say that it took nothing more than opening up a few snakes, for it was one thing to be confident that there is indeed a normal activity which is accessible to study, and quite another to actually achieve a firm understanding of that activity. The quest for such an understanding challenged some of the best minds on and off for nearly two millennia, and Harvey himself arrived at his own definitive conclusions in this regard only after many hours of often frustrating observations.[32] Moreover, through most of the preceding period it was not clear that the results of such study would shed any light at all on the issue of the movement of the blood, since it was widely assumed that the heartbeat is basically an aerating mechanism.[33] This idea is already apparent in the anonymous treatise just mentioned, it was the basic assumption of Galen and Vesalius, and as Harvey complained in De motu cordis it was still the view of his own teacher Fabricius.[34]

Still, the heartbeat provided the best entree into the inner workings of the body, and if one were to examine Harvey's discovery as a strictly physiological achievement, this is where the emphasis would necessarily lie.[35] One would need to consider, in particular, how the heartbeat came to be understood as a means to transmit blood, largely as a consequence of the discovery of the pulmonary transit in the sixteenth century; how various individuals, notably Harvey himself, arrived at a clear grasp of precisely how the heart transmits blood through its movement; and how Harvey eventually extended the sway of the heartbeat over the whole of the movement of the blood, through the theory of circulation. Indeed, he himself could epitomize his achievement by declaring, "It has been demonstrated that a perpetual movement of the blood in a circle is caused by the beat of the heart,"[36] and it was also this relationship that he had in mind when he entitled his treatise *On the Movement of the Heart and Blood in Animals.*

This side of the story having to do with the movement of the heart was clearly of crucial importance, and it will be impossible to avoid telling at least part of it in what follows. However, my principal object is to try to approach Harvey's discovery from the perspective of earlier ideas about the movement of the blood, which means in effect to try to put it into the context of pathological and therapeutic thinking, where most previous ideas about this subject were to be found. Part of the aim is to explore the problematic issues already indicated, that is, to show how certain deep-seated convictions about what is abnormal must have made it extraordinarily difficult for Harvey to arrive at a concept of the circulation as a constant, normal function. However, I also hope to show that the discovery itself was not just a matter of these old attitudes being swept aside by the results of specialized physiological investigation. It was, of course, partly that, as I have just indicated, but we shall see that in expanding his understanding of the heartbeat into the theory of circulation, Harvey was also positively aided by the very medical context which, in other respects, was so troublesome. He not only drew important inferences from various abnormal phenomena such as the haemorrhage, but also employed methods of reasoning derived from humoral pathology and therapy, and even used older pathological theories as models for the new physiological theory of circulation. Indeed, this relationship between the normal and the abnormal was probably an overt and overriding issue at the time of discovery, which consisted in significant measure in translating some of the old conceptions of abnormality into a new conception of normality. Accordingly, Harvey himself seems to have seen his theory as subsuming rather than overthrowing the old medicine, although others did not see it that way.[37]

The Hippocratics

Since many of the thought patterns that we shall be examining were first established by the Hippocratic physicians, it will be useful to begin with a few simple ideas which are found in their writings. There is, of course, no single theory of disease common to all of the diverse treatises in the Hippocratic corpus, but a basic supposition found in many of them is that disease is due to changes in one or more of several bodily fluids or humors, including notably the blood.[38] The problem might be due to a general excess or qualitative corruption of the humors, but it might also have a more local focus. To account for such localized diseases, the Hippocratic authors relied on the notion of the "flux," or forceful movement of humors to a particular part, which might result either in swelling and inflammation, or in some abnormal discharge.[39] For example,

The haemorrhoidal disease comes about in this way: bile or phlegm enfixes itself in the veins of the rectum, and it heats the blood in those veins. The veins, being heated, draw blood from the nearby veins, and the veins being filled, there is swelling of the interior of the rectum.[40]

The Hippocratic physicians seem to have regarded any external wound as having an effect analogous to the bile or phlegm in the rectal veins, i.e., as provoking a flux of blood to the site of the injury.[41] One result of this flux might be haemorrhage, but another might be inflammation, due to the abnormal aggregation of blood in the vicinity of the wound. Thus while it was important to try to staunch the external bleeding, this had to be done so as not to result in the blood simply collecting around the wound and causing inflammation. Accordingly, in addition to local treatment efforts were directed at diverting the flux away from the site of the wound through procedures such as fomentation carried out at some remote part of the body. Furthermore, to eliminate blood which had already accumulated near the wound it was advisable to let it bleed for a time, and in the case of an old wound which had become inflamed it might even be useful to reactivate the bleeding to evacuate the peccant material.

By the same reasoning, bleeding might be deliberately induced in order to relieve the effects of a flux originally stemming from purely internal causes. For example, one Hippocratic author stated that in cases of swelling and inflammation arising spontaneously, without injury, "an influx of blood into the veins is the cause."[42] Therefore, "blood is to be abstracted, especially from the veins, which are the seat of the influx, if they be conspicuous; but if not, deeper and more numerous scarifications are to be made in the swellings." However, if the flux has settled in some part that is inaccessible to such treatment, then a strategy must be adopted which induces the humor to move to some place from which it can be evacuated. For example,

In cases where phlegm is confined between the midriff and the stomach, causing pain because it has no outlet into either of the cavities, the disease is removed if the phlegm be diverted by way of the veins into the bladder.[43]

Presumably this would be accomplished by means of a diuretic, while in other cases one might choose a laxative or emetic.

However, bleeding could also be used to accomplish such remote evacuations, as explained by one of the Hippocratic authors:

Bleeding then should be practised according to these principles. The habit should be cultivated of cutting as far as possible from the places where the pains are wont to occur and the blood to collect. In this way the change will be least sudden and violent, and you will change the habit so that the blood no longer collects in the same place.[44]

Thus on the one hand external bleeding might be the result of accidental injury which provokes an unwanted flux of blood to the site, or on the other hand it might be deliberately induced in order to divert a flux from some other part. Hence the seeming paradox that bleeding might even be induced in one part of the body in order to stop an unwanted haemorrhage in some other part![45]

Further underscoring the conception of bloodletting as a means to manipulate the humoral movements is the statement of another author concerning an ancillary procedure: "In venesections, ligatures set the blood in motion, but tight ones hinder the blood."[46] As a simple description of the differing consequences of moderate and tight ligation this statement is quite unobjectionable, and in its causal implications it conforms to the more pervasive assumption that the movement of the blood is highly susceptible to provocation, with the results being either pathogenic or therapeutic according to circumstance.

Besides the more or less localized fluxes just discussed, the early Greek physicians also assumed that more generalized changes in the distribution of blood can occur under various circumstances. For example, Alcmaeon of Croton (5th century B.C.) is reported to have held that "sleep results from the inward retreat of the blood to the bloodstreaming veins and waking from its dispersal, but its complete inward retreat leads to death."[47] According to one of the Hippocratic authors this inward retreat could become a massive rush of blood to the brain should a sleeping person happen to have a frightening dream, "just as in the waking state the face is flushed, and the eyes are red, mostly when a man is afraid and his mind contemplates some evil act."[48] Another author invoked the analogy of fear to account for the fact that in the cold stage of febrile paroxysm, "the blood leaps from the extremities of the body to the viscera," with the result that "some parts of the body become over-full, but others depleted of blood."[49]

On the other hand, by a judicious choice of remedies, the physician might also achieve a high degree of control over the general distribution of humors through the body. For example, the author of *Regimen II* recommended this treatment for a patient suffering from excessive dryness of the flesh: he should be bathed, given a soft wine to drink, and then allowed to eat and drink his fill; "then he should let a longish interval pass, until the veins become filled and inflated. Then let him vomit, and, having gone a short stroll, sleep on a soft bed."[50] The author then explained that the effect of this treatment would be to moisten the dried body, but without causing an excess:

For the body, in a state of dryness, after the entrance of all sorts of food, draws to itself what is beneficial from the several foods for the several parts of the body; on being filled and moistened, the belly having been emptied by the emetic, it casts away the excess, while the belly, being empty, exercises a revulsion. So the flesh rejects the excessive moisture, but it does not cast away that which is of an appropriate amount, unless it be under the constraint of drugs, of exercises, or of some revulsion.[51]

Thus by the bath, the wine, and the copious feeding, the physician hopes to promote a general movement of nutriment outward through the veins; then by the emetic, the stroll, and the sleep, he seeks to reverse the process, leaving the body well nourished, but not burdened by an excess.

This passage brings us the closest that we have come so far to what might be called the physiology of humoral flow, i.e., an indication of what happens under normal circumstances, in the absence of pathological or therapeutic disruption. It comes down simply to this, that food is consumed, digested in the belly, distributed by the veins, and absorbed by the various parts of the body in amounts appropriate to their needs. Such assumptions seem fairly widespread in the Hippocratic writings, but are usually mentioned only in passing, with little elaboration beyond these bare essentials.[52]

Galen

In post-Hippocratic medicine the interest in physiology became much more considerable, a development that was closely related to the growth of general natural philosophy, on the one hand, and animal and human anatomy, on the other. Galen, for instance, devoted an entire treatise, *On the Natural Faculties,* to developing the physiology of nutrition that was passed over so lightly by most of his Hippocratic forebears. He outlined a precise anatomical pathway for the food—from gut through portal veins, liver, and systemic veins to the body at large—and sought to define the varying roles of the organs situated along this pathway in concocting the food and eliminating waste substances. He also invoked the principles of natural philosophy to analyze the underlying nature of the changes from food to blood, and from blood to tissue. Above all, he sought to establish that every part of the body must have four inherent teleological powers or faculties, whereby it *attracts* food of the proper kind and amount, *retains* it for an appropriate period of time, *assimilates* it to its own substance, and *expels* whatever is qualitatively or quantitatively useless to it.[53]

However, while Galen did devote considerable intellectual effort to the elaboration of this theory, in its broad essentials it did not go much beyond the recognition by the Hippocratic physicians that men and animals must be nourished, and that the nourishment must be distributed from the digestive organs to all the parts of the body. Furthermore, one need only examine some of Galen's many pathological treatises to see that in his own mind the value of the doctrine of natural faculties lay as much in providing a theoretical foundation for Hippocratic doctrines as in explaining the normal process of nutrition.[54]

Indeed, in Galen's view the disruption of the nutritive process at one stage or another was the most fundamental mechanism in the causation of internal disease. Thus a general humoral disruption might result from the consumption of too much or the wrong kind of food, or from a disorder of a central concocting organ such as the stomach or liver. If the consequence is a simple excess of blood that is otherwise healthy it is called "plethora," while if the qualitative composition of the blood is faulty, the state is one of "cacochymia" (literally, "bad humors").[55] However, the problem may be confined to a single organ, based on some local disturbance of the natural faculties. For example, a failure of the expulsive faculty of some part will result in a flux, which is nothing more than the collection around the affected part of the wastes expelled by other parts.[56] The immediate consequence is local plenitude or swelling, but if the part does not succeed either in assimilating or in expelling the excess, putrefaction will develop, leading to inflammation.[57] Inflammation, in turn, brings with it an increase of heat as well as pain, and both of the latter have the effect of positively attracting additional material to the part, thus making things all the worse.[58]

Galen also envisioned various ways in which general and local conditions might interact to produce more complex disease mechanisms.[59] For example, a state of general plethora or cacochymia increases the need for all parts to expel excessive or harmful substances from themselves, and so it is under such conditions that a flux to a relatively weak part is especially likely to occur.[60] On the other hand, localized inflammation can have systemic effects if, for instance, the heat and pain become so great that there is a general movement of blood to the site, causing chills in the rest of the body.[61] These are just a few relatively simple examples to show how, through his theory of natural faculties, Galen had devised not only a comprehensive explanation of the physiology of nutrition, but also a pathological theory of great flexibility.

However, to account for rapid changes in blood distribution through the whole body Galen found it convenient to resort to an additional hypothesis, based upon the Stoic doctrine of tonic motion. The Stoics had postulated a fine material *pneuma* or spirit that pervades the whole Cosmos, and undergoes a constant movement of *tonos* or tension.[62] This motion was described by one ancient author as follows:

Cohesion is a spirit ever returning to itself. It begins to extend itself from the center of the body in question to its extremes, and when it has reached the outermost surface it reverses its course, till it arrives at the place from which it first set out. This regular double course of cohesion is indestructible; and it is this which runners imitate at the triennial festivals.[63]

As this statement suggests, the pneuma and its tonic movement are the basis for cohesion in every individual object. Additionally, they provide for nutrition in plants, sensation in animals, and, on the cosmic level, for sympathy among all things. Furthermore, the Stoics looked to disruptions in the balance between inward and outward movement to account for various disturbances in these functions.[64] Sleep, for example, is a temporary inward collapse of the *tonos,* resulting in the deadening of the senses. Similarly, strong emotions were viewed as "perturbations" of the pneuma, with either inward or outward movement gaining the upper hand.

Galen adopted this basic concept from the Stoics, although he applied it to the innate heat of the body rather than the pneuma. In his view, this heat is identical with nature and soul,

so that if you understand its substance to be self-moved and ever-in-motion you will not be wrong. . . . And in its ceaseless motion the innate heat does not only move inward or outward, but one of these movements always succeeds the other. For if it relaxed only inward it would quickly cease to move, but if it moved only outward it would be dissipated and so perish on that account.[65]

Galen made some effort to give this doctrine a general physiological significance, especially by relating it to his theory of respiration, but it appears that its chief interest for him was to account for various unusual phenomena, which often involved movements of the blood as well.[66] As he put it, "the inward and outward tendency of the innate heat gives rise to many perturbations of the soul; and along with the heat, spirit and blood are at times borne inward and contracted to their source, at other times expand outward and are diffused."[67] As a prime example of the evident movement of heat, spirit, and blood to the inner regions of the body Galen cited the emotion fear, while anger was his archetype of outward dispersal. Joy involves a more moderate outward movement, and sadness a less strenuous inward movement. Shame is a compound process, beginning with movement to the inner regions, followed by rapid movement to the exterior. The causes of such movements may also be physical, rather than psychological. Taking a hot bath, for example, will result in the movement of the blood to the periphery of the body, while a cold bath causes inward revocation. And vigorous exercise sets up simultaneous inward and outward movements, although eventually the outward movement gains the upper hand, resulting in fatigue.

These inward and outward movements are not necessarily dangerous, but in Galen's view they always had the potentiality of being so. Conditions such as anger or prolonged exercise, which cause blood to flow to the outer parts, can mimic the symptoms of plethora (i.e., an absolute excess of blood), and if carried to an extreme can even give rise to fever.[68] On the other hand, sudden fear can result in death in those who are weak by nature, "because the blood comes together and is carried to the principle," where it has a suffocating effect.[69] However, according to Galen no one has ever died from anger, although some weak-souled individuals do succumb to excessive joy.

While inward and outward movements of heat and blood can thus have pathogenic results, they can in turn come about in consequence of other pathological conditions. For example, in certain kinds of ephemeral fevers "a hot but sweet humor is borne from the depths of the body to the skin, . . . so that in such patients the face appears quite florid, and somewhat swollen."[70] And if the fever is an intermittent one, the paroxysm will involve both inward and outward movement in sequence. According to Galen the tertian fever comes about when some part becomes inflamed and periodically discharges putrid bile to the whole body (if the humor were black bile the fever would be quartan, while phlegm would result in a quotidian).[71] The bile passes out of the veins into the sentient parts of the body, which then try to rid themselves of the noxious humor through their expulsive faculties.[72] However, before they can accomplish this the bile has a recoiling effect on the blood and innate heat. As Galen put it,

At this time the blood, and with it the innate heat, contracts to the inner regions of the body, and to the viscera, leaving cold and bloodless the parts near the skin and the extremities, which are remote from the viscera. If the innate heat were to be extinguished or suffocated within the depths of the body, . . . the animal would die.[73]

If all goes well, however, this inward gathering of heat and blood is simply a prelude to an all-out assault on the bile:

But after taking refuge in the inner parts [the innate heat] gather itself together to resist the offending cause. It thus becomes like a tool for the expulsive faculty that is resident in all parts of the body. This faculty by itself was intended to expel noxious substances, but it does so much more effectively with the aid of the innate heat, which now expands outward from the inner parts, and, by the vehemence of its motion, expels the material to whatever place is most convenient. Usually the peccant material is expelled through the skin, but often through vomiting or from the bowels.[74]

Thus the cold, the hot, and the sweating stage of the malarial paroxysm are interpreted as a sequence of inward and outward movements by the heat and blood.

In Galen's view, then, the blood can undergo countless patterns of movement in response to changing circumstances, but while many of these movements are harmful, the medical practitioner in turn has considerable powers to intervene and change the humoral movements for the better. For example, if an individual is suffering from emaciation, one should counteract it not only by providing a plentiful diet, but by heat, exercise, massage, and other such measures as will cause redness and swelling. As Galen put it, "the object of such measures is, by attracting good blood into the fleshy substance, to strengthen the nutritive faculty therein, in order that what is attracted may not be eliminated."[75] If only a certain part of the body is suffering a deficit of food, then localized fomentation and massage should be used.[76]

More often than not, however, the problem would be one of counteracting an excess of material flowing to some part. Various procedures were available for this purpose, but they generally fell into two broad categories, namely derivation and revulsion.[77] Derivation would be used when it appeared that a humoral flux was largely completed, leaving an existing state of local plenitude that had to be relieved. In this case the procedure would be carried out as close to the part as possible, with the aim of directly evacuating the harmful excess. On the other hand, revulsive therapy would be employed when it was determined that a flux was still in progress, and could thus be prevented from reaching its presumed target. In this case the procedure would be carried out at a site remote from the threatened organ, in order to divert the flux away from the latter. For example, just as local fomentation and massage might be used for the positive purpose of drawing extra blood to the site of application, so might they be used to draw humors away from some other part threatened with an excess. In other cases the aim would be not just to shift the patterns of flow within the body, but to evacuate the diverted material through some form of purgation, such as a clyster or an emetic.

For Galen the haemorrhage fitted into this set of assumptions in two ways. He had learned to distinguish clearly between the arterial and the venous haemorrhage, but much like the Hippocratics he looked upon the escape of blood in either case largely as the consequence of a flux that was provoked by the infliction of the wound.[78] If this were the unwanted result of trauma the aim of therapy would be to stop the flow of blood, and the means to do this would include procedures carried out on remote parts of the body in order to revulse the flow away from the wound.[79] However, by the same reasoning the deliberately induced haemorrhage (venesection) was viewed as a powerful means to revulse or derive an internal flux, or even to stem an unwanted haemorrhage.[80] It might also be used to relieve plethora, or a general excess of blood in the whole body,[81] but plethora itself could affect some parts more than others, so that often the evacuation was quite specifically targeted. As Galen explained, cutting open a given vein will to some extent evacuate the whole body, but it will evacuate some parts more quickly and to a much greater extent than others, so that it is very important to know which vein to choose to alleviate a given part.[82] In pleuritis, for example, the opening of the internal cubital vein will evacuate the site of the inflammation much more extensively than it will the rest of the body.[83]

Galen was also familiar with various ways in which ligatures might be used to control the movement of the blood, both to stimulate and to inhibit. He knew the Hippocratic dictum that "in venesection, ligatures set the blood in motion, but tight ones hinder the blood," and added that other means to promote the flow of blood in venesection include heating, massaging, and exercising the part of the body, thus showing that he placed the moderately tight ligature into the category of things which promote the flow of blood toward the site of application.[84] Accordingly, he also advocated the use of such ligatures without venesection as a means to temporarily divert blood from one part of the body to another remote part.[85]

The tight ligature likewise had medical significance beyond the issue of bloodletting. Galen assumed that the effect of tight binding is to cut off the

flow of blood and heat to the affected part. This would usually be an unde-
sired side effect to be avoided in bandaging, but it might be turned to positive
advantage. For example, if a part is suffering from emaciation this might be
counteracted not only by taking steps to attract extra blood to the affected
part, but also by tightly binding a nearby healthy part in order to divert blood
away from it.[86] Galen appears not to have used external tight binding as a
means to control bleeding (i.e., the tourniquet), but he was quite familiar
with the technique of direct vascular ligation for this purpose.[87]

Ligatures also figured prominently in many of Galen's vivisectional procedures, and in some cases one can see a direct relationship between the therapeutic and the experimental applications. For example, in his treatise *On
the Usefulness of the Pulse* he maintained that the arteries play a crucial role
in sustaining the heat of the body, and that the veins also do so to a lesser extent. As evidence for this he cited surgical experience with vascular ligation:

Sometimes it happens that veins and arteries are injured in such a way that it is
necessary for surgeons to tie them off with ligatures. And all patients to whom this is
done feel the [affected] parts become colder within a short space of time, and this happens especially quickly if both the arteries and the veins have been tied, more slowly if
only the arteries, but very little at all if only the veins.[88]

Thus the point of interest is a side effect—clearly undesirable from the
medical point of view—of the surgical procedure. However, for those who
might not have access to such surgical experience Galen went on to suggest a
deliberate experiment:

Indeed, if you want to apply a very tight ligature to some part of the body without any
wound, you will immediately see that it is rendered livid and cold, clearly because it
has been deprived of the heat which flows from within to all the parts of the body.[89]

In this case Galen was interested in the perception of heat loss by the
subject, and therefore it was necessary to rely on human beings who had
either been accidentally wounded, or on whom an experiment was performed
without injury. In other cases, however, the function under consideration was
directly perceptible by the operator, and therefore the way was open for
deliberate animal vivisection, involving direct vascular ligation, either singly
or in combination with other procedures. Simplest of all, perhaps, was the
direct ligation of an exposed artery to demonstrate the loss of pulse in the
distal portion.[90] However, this could then be elaborated in various ways, both
to provide further insights into the underlying cause of the pulse and to shed

light on the question of whether the arteries normally contain blood.[91] Similarly, Galen described a wide variety of procedures involving the direct ligation and section of nerves and the spinal cord, in order to demonstrate the role of these organs in sensation and voluntary movement.[92]

Galen also discussed the experimental ligation of veins, but chiefly to point out that it produces no dramatic effect comparable to that which results from the tying of arteries and nerves. As he put it,

> If nerves are interrupted by a ligature, or severed, those parts continuous with the brain can be seen to retain their faculties, but those parts beyond the ligature immediately lose both sense and movement. So too with the arteries, those continuous with the heart retain their original faculties, but those cut off by the ligature immediately cease to pulsate....[However], if you similarly interrupt the vein extending to some part with a ligature, or even cut it out entirely, the part will become emaciated and discolored over some prolonged period, but it will not suffer any immediate harm worth mentioning.[93]

Galen attributed this difference to the inherently tranquil, plant-like character of the nutritive process, and he had no doubt that through anatomical evidence he could prove quite conclusively that the blood does indeed move slowly outward through the veins to nourish the body.

From our perspective, the most striking feature of this account is Galen's failure to take note of any swelling of the veins distal to the ligature, but such an effect would have been quite irrelevant to the avowed aim of the experiment. The latter was explicitly modelled on the ligation of nerves and arteries, in which some function that is clearly present before the procedure is eliminated in consequence of it. These were, in effect, exercises in experimental pathology, so that the kind of result that Galen expected was paralysis or emaciation, rather than a positive response such as muscular contraction or distal venous swelling.[94]

It was probably for much the same reason that Galen apparently did not try to draw any physiological conclusions from the effects of the moderately tight ligature applied to an uninjured limb, in contrast to his use of the tight ligature to demonstrate the influx of heat, as discussed above. Galen did, however, employ the moderate ligature for a different kind of investigative purpose, namely to make the veins more accessible to study. In his treatise on the anatomy of the veins and arteries, he noted that the superficial veins of the arm "can be clearly seen in thin human subjects even without dissection, if a ligature is applied to the arm."[95] In *On Anatomical Procedures* he gave a fuller account of a variant technique:

All these veins [in the lower arm] can be seen even without dissection in many men who are both thin and full-blooded, and have large veins, especially if the surrounding air is warm or the man just have had a bath. You must compress the part with your hand where you wish the full veins to be clearly seen. You should do this often and in many subjects.[96]

Galen's reference to heat as an additional factor in swelling the veins again underscores his assumption that the moderate ligature is a means to provoke abnormal movements of the blood, and so it is not at all surprising that he should be freely familiar with the phenomenon but not see it as having any physiological implications.

Similar considerations would have effectively excluded the use of venesection itself as a technique in physiological investigation. After all, if one routinely opens veins therapeutically with the precise intention of profoundly altering the patterns of humoral flow, one would not turn around and use the same technique in order to investigate the normal movement of the blood.

The Arterial Haemorrhage

Interestingly enough, however, Galen did devote considerable effort to the experimental opening of arteries, and even made this the subject of a special treatise, *On Whether Blood is Naturally Contained in the Arteries.* As we shall see, the conclusions that he drew from such experiments were heavily influenced by the polemical atmosphere in which they were carried out as well as by his own theoretical preconceptions. Nevertheless, the issue is of the highest interest for our present discussion, because the debate explicitly turned on the relationship between the normal and the abnormal in the realm of animal experimentation, and between pathology and physiology in the realm of medical theory.

As Galen made clear at the beginning of his treatise, both sides were in agreement that if one cuts into an artery in a living animal, blood will immediately flow out.[97] Most physicians, Galen himself included, interpreted this to mean that blood is "naturally" contained in the arteries, i.e., that it is there all along, independently of the cutting of the artery. However, the followers of Erasistratus, the great physician and anatomist of the third century B.C., viewed the outflow of blood as a fundamental distortion of the natural situation.[98] In their view the arteries normally contain only an aerial *pneuma,* while blood is confined to the venous system. Whenever an artery is cut, these conditions are disrupted, as pneuma escapes through the opening, thereby creating a vacuum within the arteries, which in turn causes blood to pass over from the veins and out through the opening, making it appear as if the blood were there all along.

At first glance, this explanation of the arterial haemorrhage might appear to be rather arbitrary, indeed obscurantist, but when viewed in the broader context of Erasistratus's medical theories it appears much less so.[99] Briefly, Erasistratus maintained that animals are subject to a steady loss of their minute constituent particles through invisible emanation, and that the two fundamental processes of nutrition and respiration serve to replace this lost substance.[100] The veins and arteries supply the body with food (blood) and air, respectively, and simple mechanical principles figure importantly in the distribution of both substances. For example, every particle that is lost by the body leaves behind a small area of vacuum, thus creating a peripheral force of attraction that draws the blood outward through the veins.[101] On the other hand, when the left ventricle of the heart dilates, it draws in air through the pulmonary veins by the power of a vacuum, and when it contracts it forcefully propels the air into the arteries, thereby causing their diastole by mechanical inflation.[102]

Furthermore, by insisting on the normal confinement of blood to the veins the Erasistrateans could then look to its abnormal passage into the arteries as a fundamental principle of pathology.[103] Thus, if the amount of food consumed exceeds the amount of bodily substance lost through invisible emanation, then the result is plethora, or an excess of blood in the veins. As this excess mounts up it will first fill the veins to capacity, then distend them beyond their usual proportions, and finally spill over into the arteries through minute anastomoses connecting the two kinds of vessel.[104] The presence of blood in the larger arteries will, in turn, interfere with the currents of pneuma flowing out from the heart, thereby causing fever. And as the pneumatic currents persist they will compact the blood into the smallest arterial branches, thus resulting in inflammation. The passage of blood from arteries into veins will also result from any external injury, since this is bound to open some arterial branches, however small, and cause a loss of pneuma.[105] The resulting vacuum in the arteries will be refilled by the entrance of blood from the veins, just as under normal conditions the blood from the veins is drawn into the empty spaces of the tissues. The opening itself may soon be healed, but once the blood has entered the arteries it can again be impacted by the continuing pneumatic currents, and so give rise to inflammation in the vicinity of the cut.

Whether the original cause of the transfusion was general plethora or local trauma, the basic aim of therapy was to induce the blood to move back from the arteries into the veins. This in turn required a diminution in the amount of blood in the veins, since according to Erasistratus "veins which are evacuated will more easily receive the blood which has spilled over into the arteries."[106] To accomplish this Erasistratus recommended placing the patient on a starvation diet. In addition, for wounds or localized inflammation the Erasistrateans advocated various revulsive techniques which would draw the blood away from the affected part, and also promote its passage back into the veins.[107]

Thus the efforts by the Erasistrateans to show that the arterial haemorrhage is a totally abnormal phenomenon were indeed aimed at protecting their doctrines, but there was nothing arbitrary about their proffered explanation, since it was quite in accordance with their general physiological, pathological, and therapeutic principles. In effect, they dismissed the arterial haemorrhage as abnormal not simply because it was embarrassing to their theories, but because it corresponded in a fundamental way with what they regarded as abnormal.

Galen vehemently opposed this explanation of the flow of blood from arteries, but he did so in large measure because he rejected the broad principles of Erasistratean medicine, and not because he necessarily had a greater respect for brute facts. He not only held that the distribution and assimilation of food are governed by the four natural faculties of attraction, retention, assimilation, and expulsion, and not by mechanical principles, he further held that there is in the heart a special faculty that causes both the heart and all the arteries to undergo constant, active pulsatile movement, which serves primarily to ventilate the innate heat throughout the body.[108] The presence of blood in the arteries was of no great importance in Galen's theoretical system, but what moved him to advocacy of this position seems to have been the particular importance which he attached to this notion of active arterial pulsation. For the Erasistrateans themselves had acknowledged that the normal presence of blood in the arteries would block the free flow of the pneuma and therefore be inconsistent with their mechanical interpretation of the pulse, so that by establishing that blood is indeed normally present Galen could greatly strengthen his own view that the pulse is an active movement caused by a special faculty.[109]

However, in attempting to devise such a demonstration Galen was constrained by the cunning of the Erasistratean position, which held that any effort to open an artery to determine its contents would automatically create the conditions under which it would contain blood.[110] Consequently, Galen's main tactic was to try to reduce Erasistratus's explanation of the arterial haemorrhage to a kind of quantitative absurdity.[111] Galen asserted that, on the Erasistratean theory, it could not just be a particular wounded artery that loses its pneuma and becomes filled with blood, but that all the pneuma from the entire arterial system would have to rush to the cut artery and out through the opening. Only when the most remote arteries had yielded their pneuma to the ones closer to the opening would blood begin to flow in from the veins to replace the pneuma, and the blood would reach the punctured artery last of all, on the heels of the last portion of escaping pneuma. "And so," said Galen, "all the blood in the entire body would flow to the cut. And this is indeed the case, for we see that from any one artery (as long as it is of some appreciable size), unless you suppress the flow, all the blood from the entire body rushes out."[112] Now to account for this fact on the Erasistratean theory, we must suppose that "all the pneuma" in the arteries rushes out through even the smallest opening without our perceiving it; following this "the whole of the blood" must pass from the veins into the arteries, and finally out through the opening; and all of this must happen so quickly that we perceive no delay between the puncturing of the artery and the outrush of blood![113] Thus we must make absurd and drastic assumptions in order to explain something so simple as the fact that blood immediately flows out of an artery upon our puncturing it. How much more reasonable, Galen argued, to suppose that the blood was there all along.

When we look beyond this obvious disagreement, however, we find that Galen's further assumptions about the presence of blood in the arteries were not really all that different from those of his opponents. Galen accepted the notion of minute arterio-venous anastomoses that Erasistratus had postulated, and maintained that every time the arteries actively dilate, a potential vacuum is created which would tend to draw in blood from the veins.[114] He also held that when the arteries contract, they return blood, heat, and pneuma back to the veins through the same anastomoses. In effect Galen took the Erasistratean pathogenic-therapeutic sequence, in which blood passes from veins into arteries, and is then induced to flow back again, and transformed it into a constant physiological process, occurring every time the arteries actively dilate and contract. Moreover, Galen freely acknowledged that he was indeed translating Erasistratean pathology into his own physiology.[115] He argued that if Erasistratus were correct on the existence of the arterio-venous connections (and Galen agreed that he was), then he would also have to admit that Nature created those pathways because she intended that blood should normally pass from the veins into the arteries. Otherwise, he would be forced to the teleologically absurd conclusion that Nature had endowed men and animals with structures which served no useful purpose, but which could cause serious harm. In other words, in Galen's view there could be no inherently pathogenic processes in nature; disease can of course occur, but only through the disruption of inherently beneficial physiological processes.

Consistent with this outlook, Galen could maintain that blood normally passes from veins into arteries, and from arteries back to veins, but also acknowledge that it can do so in increased amounts under unusual circumstances. He himself argued that the passage occurs so readily that plethora within the veins usually does result in an extra overflow to the arteries.[116] Furthermore, he endorsed the dictum of Erasistratus that "veins which are evacuated will more easily receive the blood which has spilled over into the arteries," but criticized him for not recognizing that venesection was a much safer and more efficient way of accomplishing this than placing the patient on a starvation diet.[117]

Thus for Galen too the passage of blood from veins into arteries had its abnormal aspects, and when we look more closely at his understanding of the arterial haemorrhage we find that such considerations were very much in evidence here as well. In the discussions cited above, he pointed to the flow of blood from the arteries simply to prove its normal presence there, but in several other places he examined the phenomenon with an eye toward establishing that the means of entry is through the arterio-venous anastomoses. For example, in *On the Usefulness of the Pulse* he reported:

If someone takes an animal of a kind which has large and manifest veins and arteries, ... or even a human being, and wounds many of its large arteries, all the blood of the animal will be exhausted through them. Let us therefore make trial of this matter: and when we always find the veins evacuated together with the arteries, we will be persuaded of the truth of the doctrine about the common openings of veins and arteries, and of the common transit from one into the other through them. Indeed, through these transits the dilated arteries draw from the veins and when contracted expel into them.[118]

However, if Galen used the demonstration to vindicate his physiological doctrine of mutual exchanges, it is just as apparent that he regarded the experiment as involving grossly pathological aspects as well. For under normal conditions the uptake of blood from the veins is matched by a return, so that at any given time most of the body's blood remains within the veins. When arteries are opened, however, the mutual exchange is somehow converted to a one-way evacuation, so that all of the blood from the veins is soon taken up by the arteries and expelled through the opening. Thus Galen's disagreement with the Erasistrateans concerning the normality of the phenomenon did not extend much beyond the first portion of blood that is expelled immediately after opening the arteries—once that has been evacuated, there follows a massive movement from veins into arteries that bears no relationship to the normal order of things. Indeed, while the simple issue of the presence of blood in the arteries was the subject of explicit controversy regarding its normality or abnormality, it apparently did not even occur to Galen that the massiveness of the evacuation could represent anything but a profoundly abnormal movement.

More generally, it seems fair to say that the net effect of Galen's physiological, pathological, and therapeutic doctrines was to place the normal movement of the blood beyond the realm of direct experimental investigation, since the techniques available, such as the ligation and sectioning of vessels, would themselves be looked upon as the primary cause of any movements which they revealed. In saying this, however, I do not mean to suggest that Galen indulged in deliberate obscurantism, i.e., that he was consciously aware that certain phenomena were threatening to his physiological doctrines and therefore had to be placed into the limbo of experimental artifact. Rather, it was a much subtler process, in which Galen's genuinely held convictions about what is normal and what is abnormal served as a constant point of reference in interpreting the phenomena relating to the movement of the blood which he encountered in the course of his medical and surgical practice, and of his animal vivisections.

The Renaissance

Galenic medicine was, of course, the common heritage of all European physicians from the Middle Ages through Harvey's day and beyond. Since long before Harvey, individual aspects of Galen's doctrine were subject to challenge or outright rejection, but some basic elements seemed almost beyond question: humoral pathology, for example, the theory of natural faculties, the importance of dietetic regulation (the non-naturals), the value of therapeutic bloodletting. These were the sorts of things over which there might be endlesss disagreements regarding specific application, but not over the fundamental principles, which seemed to be self-evidently true.

Among these universally shared convictions was the notion that the movement of the blood is an extremely volatile activity, subject to the most profound alterations in response to a broad range of circumstances. Many of these fluxes would be local in character, but in the views of Renaissance physicians, as for Galen, the blood, along with the heat and spirits, could also be provoked into massive inward or outward movements. These processes of "expansion" and "concentration," as they were called, were associated with a wide variety of phenomena, including sleep and waking, blushing and pallor of the skin, the swelling and subsidence of peripherial veins, increases or diminutions of the pulse, palpitations of the heart, sweating, chills, fever, invigoration, fainting, weakness, numbness, torpor, and sudden death. They might arise from any number of causes, including diseases, vigorous exercise, strong emotions such as fear, anger, joy, sorrow, and shame, external heat and cold, and medical procedures such as ligatures, cupping, bloodletting, and massage.

Harvey's more immediate predecessors were also familar with the general principle of tonic movement from which Galen had derived such unusual events, although as a physiological principle this continued to be relatively lacking in specific content. For example, in 1626 a Paduan medical professor named Pompeio Caimo published a treatise on the innate heat, in which he declared:

The innate spirit..., as a compound of fire and air, undergoes perennial motion, so ordered that it takes place from the center to the circumference, and from the circumference back to the center, and as long as this persists there is a kind of movement from the same point and to the same point, since it begins from the center and ends in the center.[119]

Caimo made a valiant attempt to explain what this meant as a physiological principle, although the whole discussion remained at a rather abstract level.[120]

By contrast, Giovanni Argenterio managed to achieve a balance between concreteness and generality in his treatise *On Sleep and Waking*, published in 1556. Argenterio's basic thesis was that rapid inward concentration of the innate heat deadens the sense organs and causes sleep, while its rapid outward expansion results in waking.[121] He made it quite clear, however, that heat itself is only a quality, and therefore incapable of undergoing such movements apart from the blood and spirits in which it inheres.[122] As evidence for his contention, he noted:

During waking the face and other external parts are red, and well colored, each according to its nature; but they become pale and livid during sleep, which could only happen because at this time all the blood, or at least its lighter and more spirituous portion, betakes itself to the inner parts, while in waking it rushes out to the external parts.[123]

This theory also accords with the assumption that many other general affections of the body are due to rapid inward and outward movements of heat:

We see that in weaknesses of the mind, fear, dread, anger, joy, sadness, febrile rigors and the subsequent hot stage, and other universal passions of soul and body which have a rapid and nearly instantaneous onset and termination—all of these occur by the power and movement of this heat, so that it is reasonable that sleep and waking should have the same cause.[124]

Accordingly, Argenterio's analysis of sleep provided the occasion to review these many other circumstances in which concentration or expansion of heat, blood, and spirits occur.

Argenterio maintained that these continuing shifts in the distribution of heat are not haphazard, but reflect the changing activities of the many individual parts of the body which use the heat as their instruments. As he stated:

It is easy to show that all actions occur by movement of the inflowing heat, that is, of blood and spirit. For we see that through waking, thinking, massages, baths, hot air, and many other factors, such substance is impelled to the surface of the body. . . . And the heat is recalled to the inner regions, and subserves those parts, during sleep, idleness, and inactivity. But through exercises it is propelled equally both inward and outward, so that it imparts its power to the entire body.[125]

However, while Argenterio attempted to place these shifts of heat and blood into an overall teleological framework, he recognized that they could also have undesirable consequences. For example, in anger "the heart itself is agitated, and the blood and spirits contained in it are heated up and expelled to the entire body, so that the individual parts become red and inflamed, because of the hot blood that is transmitted."[126] Even more dramatically, "we see that in such an affection of the heart [as great joy] the blood and spirits are moved outward, so that sometimes men die as a result of the heat deserting the internal viscera."[127]

Accordingly, the subjects of expansion and concentration were also topics of prime interest in specialized monographs on diseases of the heart, such as that published by Hannibal Albertini, in the early seventeenth century. In his view, whenever such emotions as anger, joy, sorrow, cares, anxiety, and worry occur, "the spirits, running here and there, now from the center to the circumference, now on the contrary from the circumference to the center, become heated, and when the heat has been communicated to the heart, there occurs palpitation of the heart."[128] Palpitation might also be due to plethora, a general excess of blood which engorges the ventricles of the heart, but "the same can occur without plethora, in sudden and great fear, in which all the blood flows into the ventricles of the heart because of its attractive faculty, and produces the varied, unequal, and disordered beats of palpitation."[129] Similarly, according to Albertini, "in every syncope [fainting] there occurs the aggregation of blood and spirits around the heart."[130]

Strong emotions were not the only cause of potentially dangerous concentrations, for according to Albertini "the same can happen at the beginnings of febrile accessions, when blood suddenly flows from the whole external surface to the internal viscera, whence compressions and obstructions occur, with danger of suffocation of the innate heat of the heart."[131] In the complete sequence of the febrile paroxysm, however, this inward concentration would be followed by outward expansion, whose effect would be salutary. Ercole Sassonia, who was professor of practical medicine at the University of Padua in the early seventeenth century, reflected the views of Galen in this regard:

In the beginning of the accession [of the intermittent paroxysm] the humors move from the circumference to the center; during the increase, from the center to the circumference; during the height, strongly from the center to the circumference; and during the decline [the humors] are digested, or are evacuated through insensible vapors, or through sweats.[132]

Sassonia's discussion also reflects an interesting point of terminology regarding intermittent fevers. The Greek term for the regularly recurring cycles of such diseases was "periodos," and since antiquity this had been most commonly translated into Latin by its exact cognate "circuitus" (both mean literally "the way around").[133] Reflecting this usage, Sassonia made reference to "the causes of the circuits of intermittent fevers, why, that is, the quotidians return and repeat their accessions every day, the tertians every other day, and the quartans every third day."[134] Following Galen, he associated these circuits with putrid phlegm, bile, and melancholy, respectively, but he also maintained that "the blood itself has its proper circuits when inflammations result from the blood, which occurs for the most part because of a flux of blood from place to place." Thus Harvey's predecessors were familiar with a "circuit of the blood" (his favorite term for the circulation), but as a strictly pathological phenomenon.

Another Paduan professor with a special interest in the circuits of intermittent fever was G. T. Minadoi, who in 1602 served as the chief *promotor* for Harvey's medical degree. In 1599, shortly before Harvey's arrival in Italy, Minadoi published for the benefit of his medical students a tract *On the Cause of the Periodicity of Fevers,* in which he took up the question of why it is that putrid phlegm, bile, and melancholy should each cause a different circuit. I shall not go into the explanation which Minadoi himself advocated, but among the many opposing views which he considered was one which ascribed the differences to the relative abundance *(copia)* of the three humors: "phlegm, as more abundant than the other humors, causes a quotidian circuit; melancholy, as more meagre than the others, causes a quartan; and bile, as intermediate between the other two in amount or abundance, causes an intermediate paroxysm, that is, a tertian."[135] His objections to this theory included the point that "if the argument for assigning the cause of periodicity is to be taken from abundance *[ex copia],* then it would be necessary to suppose that the blood, which is more abundant than the other humors, would make a quotidian circuit"—a line of reasoning which anticipates, if only formally, Harvey's eventual conclusion that the blood passes through the body "in such quantity and abundance *[copia],* that it is necessary for it to be moved, in some manner, in a circuit."[136]

A final point that should be noted about these massive shifts of blood, spirits, and heat is that the physician was not without power to counteract them, especially in the case of inward concentration. According to Albertini, because syncope always involves the aggregation of blood and spirit around the heart, "therefore the extremities should be rubbed, and ligatures should be applied to the limbs" in order to counteract the process.[137] Sassonia also noted that sudden inward movement of the blood can cause suffocation, and as means to revulse the blood outward he recommended rubbing, ligatures, cupping, and clysters, as well as shouting at the patient and pulling his hair, beard, and nose.[138] From this it is especially clear to what extent Harvey's predecessors considered the movement of the blood to be subject to profound alteration by extrinsic circumstances, and in particular how much power of manipulation they attributed to the medical practitioner himself.

In these instances the point of the manipulation was to try to counteract generalized inward movement, but very often the object would be much more localized and discreet in nature. For example, beginning in the 1520s and continuing throughout the sixteenth century there raged a great controversy over how best to alleviate pleuritis through venesection.[139] In his *Letter on Bloodletting* (1539) Vesalius included a figure that helps to define some of the basic issues involved.[140] The figure is entitled "the veins nourishing the

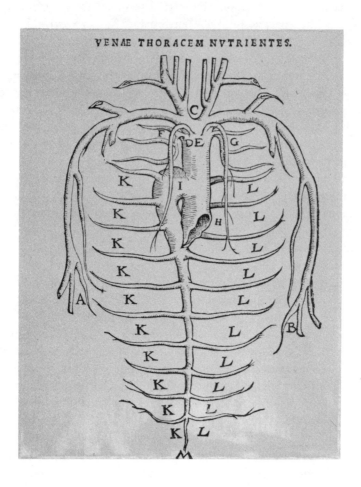

thorax," which indicates that the normal function of these vessels is simply to distribute venous blood. In a pathological context, however, they provide the field for various abnormal fluxes, including ones which can settle in some part of the thoracic wall and produce the pains associated with pleuritis. And from the therapeutic point of view, the problem then becomes one of trying to induce the peccant material to flow back through the azygos system to the vena cava, and then out through one of the arm veins to be evacuated. The point that Vesalius wished to make was that because of the asymmetry of the azygos system one should always let blood from the right arm regardless of which side of the thorax was afflicted with pain.

However, while it was important to choose the best anatomical pathway, Vesalius by no means assumed that the evacuation would be determined by structural relations alone. As he put it,

No one of sound mind would deny that the natural faculties [of the veins]...are active and involved in the process of venesection, and that the straight and transverse fibers of the veins greatly assist them in directing the flow of blood toward the wound that has been inflicted, and toward the painful ligation and friction, or toward the hot fomentation.[141]

Vesalius went on to explain further that the process of venesection is in principle identical with that of inflammation, in that Nature directs a flux of blood and spirits toward any locus of pain in an effort to repel the offending cause. During the sixteenth century various other theories were put forth to explain why blood flows out of a cut vein, but all took for granted that the movement is somehow the result of the cutting, rather than the simple release of movement occurring independently of these circumstances.[142]

A similar point of view pervaded discussions of a related therapeutic question, that of why a moderately tight ligature causes veins to swell and also promotes the escape of blood if the vein is opened. Some physicians lightly passed over the phenomenon by saying that "ligatures attract" blood,[143] but others proposed more complex causal mechanisms. For example, in a book of medical and philosophical questions published in 1523, the humanist physician Ambrogio Leone asked, "Why is it that when you tightly ligate an arm or other extremity, all the veins below the ligature immediately swell, a device which surgeons use when they are ordered to let blood?"[144] Leone was able to suggest no less than three possible reasons for this effect. One was that the distal portion of the vein is weakened by the application of the ligature, so that the excess humors of the other parts of the body tend to collect in it. Another was that the ligature initially creates a state of inanition by cutting off the flow of blood, as a result of which the veins make an unusually strong effort to draw back what they have lost, and end up with an excess. Or again,

Is it perhaps because the ligature is so annoying a thing that it stirs up the power of Nature. Nature fights against it and tries to repel it, but she can only do this by sending spirits and blood. . . . Therefore blood and spirits rush to the ligature, and by penetrating they pass through it in order to repel it. But when they have passed through they cannot return, because they are pressed by other [blood and spirit] flowing in, and therefore they accumulate greatly in the extreme veins.

Leone did not choose among these three possible mechanisms, all of which take for granted that the ligature somehow provokes a movement of blood outward to the affected vein.

Guido Guidi, the professor of surgery at the University of Pisa during the 1550s and 60s, endorsed the idea that the ligature causes pain in the part to which it is applied, and that Nature sends in a rush of blood and spirit in an effort to remove the pain.[145] In his practical directions for venesection, he pointed out that if the ligature is not tight enough, it will not cause sufficient pain to incite Nature to fill the veins, but on the other hand, it will also fail to produce swelling if it is so tight as to impede the flow of blood. Thus care had to be taken to obtain a good flow of blood in venesection and this no doubt tended to reinforce the assumption that these procedures largely create the movements of the blood which they reveal.

On the other hand, no such special steps were necessary to obtain a free flow of blood from cut arteries, although this seemed explicable on the grounds that the arteries, unlike the veins, undergo constant pulsatile movement. As Laurent Joubert explained, when arteries are cut, "they ejaculate the blood through their systole (which is their contraction), and expel it through the wound. That is, when they become narrower they compress the contained humor, and it rushes out by the exit that has been provided."[146] In addition, Joubert and his contemporaries were also quite familiar with the further point noted by Galen, that "when larger arteries have been incised, the whole of the blood is poured out, and through them is evacuated even that blood which the veins contain."[147]

Moreover, Joubert and others sometimes extended Galen's observations by noting that all the blood from both kinds of vessel can also be evacuated by opening only *veins*.[148] This interest in the passage of blood from arteries into veins probably stemmed largely from therapeutic considerations: it was generally recognized that arteriotomy is a potentially dangerous procedure, but venesection provided an alternative means of evacuating the arteries. According to Felix Platter, when it is not feasible to alleviate excess blood in the arteries by direct evacuation, "it still is quite beneficial to let blood from the veins, both to diminish the antecedent cause [i.e., the blood in the arteries is ultimately derived from the veins], and because veins which have been emptied often snatch blood from the nearby arteries."[149]

The latter assumption could also be fitted into a more elaborate therapeutic strategy. Joubert, for example, considered the question, "If febrile material is in the heart, why is it that we do not open arteries, which proceed from it, rather than veins, in order to evacuate the vicious blood which causes the disease?"[150] The answer to the first part is that it would be too dangerous to open arteries that are large enough to directly evacuate the heart. As to why the same thing can be done more safely by the opening of veins, the answer is to be found in Galen's demonstration of arterio-venous anastomoses:

But it is sufficient to let blood through the veins, because arteries and veins communicate with each other, as Galen demonstrates in *On the Usefulness of the Pulse*. For thus it happens that when veins are emptied, the arteries also become empty, and vice versa; because the mouths of these vessels are in contact with each other. Since, therefore, the heart is connected to the arteries, but the latter communicate with the veins, it is sufficient to use venesection for [evacuating] either kind of material.[151]

Thus under the right circumstances Harvey's predecessors had no difficulty in envisioning a flow of blood from heart to arteries, and from arteries over to veins, although Joubert's clear assumption is that this movement would not occur without the therapeutic intervention, which is intended precisely to stimulate such an evacuation.

Moreover, Andrea Cesalpino even described the same blood as *returning* to the heart by this pathway, and not just as part of some unusual sequence of disease and therapy, but on a routine daily basis. This was in a famous digression in his *Medical Questions* (1593), where he invoked the principle that heat and blood generally move outward from the heart during waking and inward during sleep, and then sought to specify the anatomical pathways involved.[152] Based upon the structure of the heart valves, he argued that the blood and heat must flow out from the heart through the arteries during waking, then over to the veins through the anastomoses and so back to the heart during sleep. Furthermore, in the same passage he also pointed out the fallaciousness of supposing that the moderate ligature provokes outward movement through the veins, because in that case the swelling should occur on the proximal side of the ligature. Instead, the distal swelling can only be due to a frustrated inward movement.[153] However, both from this passage and others it seems clear that Cesalpino still supposed that the usual movement of blood through the veins is outward[154]—the inward flow during sleep represents a regular reversal of the outward current, while the effect of the ligature, or of any venous blockage, is to provoke a rather forceful such reversal. Indeed, Cesalpino raised the whole subject in the first place in order to show that such a provoked inward flow through the veins can have lethal consequences if it is sufficiently massive to engorge the vessels of the thorax and cause suffocation.[155] His ideas thus provide a most graphic illustration of how the circulation could remain camouflaged under a series of presumed special effects, including the sleep cycle, the stimulant effect of the ligature, and the consequences of disease.

Similarly, a concern for the dangerous consequences of forceful outward movement of the venous blood provided Harvey's teacher Hieronymus Fabricius with a basis for explaining a new anatomic discovery, namely the existence of valve-like structures within the veins. Fabricius has frequently been criticized for his interpretation of the valves, as if he had somehow failed to see their obvious significance. However, he correctly associated the occurrence of varicose veins with the failure of the valves, and so one cannot say that he was clearly wrong in thinking that one of their major functions is to offer protection against such an occurrence.[156]

At all events, in his monograph on the venous valves, published in 1603, Fabricius proposed that their basic function is to inhibit the outward movement of the venous blood. He freely acknowledged the seeming paradox of this idea when viewed in relation to normal venous function, "for who would ever have thought that membranous valves could be found in the lumen of veins, especially as this lumen, designed for the passage of blood to the whole body, should be free for the free flow of blood."[157] However, if due regard is had for the idea that the blood must not only move outward, but do so in an appropriately tranquil and equitable manner, then it will be seen that the venous valves positively enhance the efficiency of the veins in fulfilling their assigned function:

My theory is that Nature has formed [the venous valves] to delay the blood to some extent, and to prevent the whole mass of it flooding into the feet, or hands and fingers, and collecting there. Two evils are thus avoided, namely, under-nutrition of the upper parts of the limbs, and a permanent swelling of the hands and feet. *Valves were made, therefore, to ensure a really fair general distribution of the blood for the nutrition of the various parts.*[158]

Besides demonstrating the existence of the valves, Fabricius also offered experimental proof of their function:

That the blood is indeed slowed by the valves, apart from being clear from their structure, can be tested by anyone either in the exposed veins of a cadaver, or in the living subject if he passes a ligature round the limbs as in bloodletting. For if one tries to press the blood, or to push it along by rubbing from above downwards, one will clearly see that it is intercepted and delayed by the valves.[159]

One might object that there is a vast difference between being "intercepted" and being merely "delayed," but from Fabricius's point of view the distinction was immaterial as far as the result of the streaking procedure was concerned. For following this statement he went on to note that the valves are especially important in the veins of the limbs, as protection against the body's own powers of attraction under certain circumstances:

The legs and arms are very often exercised in local movement; this movement is at times vigorous and rather violent, and in consequence vehement heat is sometimes excited within them. There is no doubt that by the power of this enkindled heat, the blood would have flowed and been attracted to the limbs in such great abundance that one of two things would have happened: either the principal [internal] organs would have been robbed of their nutriment from the vena cava, or the limb vessels would have been in danger of rupture.[160]

From this perspective, the streaking procedure would appear as just another way of placing an abnormally great burden upon the valves, a point that is underscored by a subsequent reprise of the experiment: "Indeed, anyone attempting even *with some violence* to push the blood down through the veins, would feel the resistance and power of the valves."[161] Accordingly, what the experiment showed to Fabricius was not that blood cannot move outward through the veins, but that it cannot move outward with any degree of force, whether that force comes from the body's own temporarily increased powers of attraction, or from the fingers of an experimenter streaking the vein. Under such conditions the valves snap shut, whereas under more tranquil circumstances they relax to permit the slow outward movement resulting from the body's gradual absorption of the venous blood.

Thus in Fabricius's view, the effect of the valves in the veins is to keep the venous blood in a relatively static condition. He pointed out that the arterial blood, by contrast, naturally undergoes a constant "flux and reflux," presumably resulting from the active pulsation of the arteries, which therefore have no valves because they would interfere with these normal to-and-fro movements.[162] Besides, he noted, the thickness of the tunics of the arteries makes them much more resistant than veins to disruption through excessive influx. In effect, then, Fabricius regarded the valves in the veins not so much as a physiological as an anti-pathological contrivance, and this was a view that made perfectly good sense to a medical community accustomed to think of maldistribution of blood as a major threat to health.

Spieghel on the Movement of the Heart and Blood

As a postscript to the preceding discussion, and as a prelude to our consideration of Harvey, it will be useful to examine some of the ideas of Adriaan van den Spieghel, an exact contemporary who also had a particular interest in the movement of the heart and blood.[163] Spieghel was born in Belgium in 1578, the same year as Harvey, and like him came to study under Fabricius at Padua around 1600. In 1616 he succeeded to the chair of anatomy at Padua, which was just about the same time that Harvey began his duties as lecturer on anatomy at the London College of Physicians. Spieghel died prematurely in 1625, but his principal anatomical and physiological works were published posthumously in 1626 and 1627, that is, just on the eve of the appearance of *De motu cordis.*[164]

In these works, Spieghel clearly accepted the idea that blood moves outward through both the veins and the arteries, with the venous blood serving primarily to nourish the body, and the arterial blood serving primarily to vivify.[165] However, while not denying the role of the Galenic natural faculties in distributing the blood, he showed a persistent concern with defining more powerful mechanisms to propel the blood through the body.

In the case of the arterial blood, this was no problem. Spieghel accepted the idea of pulmonary transit of the blood, and had also conducted frequent studies of the heartbeat *in vivo*. On this basis, he had concluded that the primary function of the heartbeat is:

to diffuse and impel spirituous [arterial] blood through the entire body by ceaseless motion. The blood is impelled through constriction, when the heart...drives out whatever is contained in its cavities, just as when we squeeze a sausage with our hands and propel upward and downward whatever is inside.[166]

Spieghel endorsed Galen's doctrine of active arterial pulsation, but he saw this primarily as an additional factor in propelling arterial blood outward through the body.[167]

Spieghel also felt that some comparable means would be necessary to propel the venous blood "throughout the entire body, to the upper parts as well as the lower."[168] This was the opposite side of the problem that Fabricius had raised in his monograph of the venous valves: not just how to prevent too much blood from flowing into the lower parts of the body, but how to positively promote its flow to the upper parts. Spieghel's answer was that the active pulsation of the concomitant arteries would also serve to force the venous blood outward. To confirm this view he cited the experience with ligatures in bloodletting:

This propulsion of the blood was highly necessary, since without it the blood would never reach the upper and lateral parts of the body. This is the reason why the veins are always accompanied by arteries, by virtue of which the movement of the venous blood is effected.... We learn this very fact from a clear experiment, that when the veins are tightly ligated, even if they are incised, we see that either no blood is given up at all, or else that it flows very slowly, and without impetus; but when the ligatures are afterwards relaxed, the blood spurts out with a kind of force and impulse. And this happens for no other reason than that the arteries, because they are ligated together with the veins, are completely deprived of motion; but when the ligatures are loosened, [the arteries] impel [the veins] by their motion, and pour forth the blood with a certain force.[169]

It was, of course, a matter of common knowledge that very tight binding inhibits the flow of blood in venesection and that it also cuts off the pulse, but to my knowledge Spieghel was the first to suggest a causal relationship between the two effects.

In this passage Spieghel concerned himself only with the question of what forces the blood to escape from an incised vein, but other related discussions included the further question of where the escaping blood comes from. Here he simply took for granted the standard assumptions of therapeutic bloodletting: in some cases it is a matter of blood actually flowing from the arteries through the anastomoses, into the veins and out through the opening, but usually it is a matter of the arteries squeezing out blood which has flowed from the central into the peripheral veins.[170]

However, while some outward propulsion of the venous blood is quite beneficial, too much of it might not be. To prevent this Spieghel looked to the valves in the veins, which he described as facing inward toward the trunk of the vena cava. Like his mentor Fabricius he saw their function as being to *regulate* rather than to *prevent* outward venous flow, noting in particular that "in the manner of valves they interrupt the pathway of the blood that rushes impetuously during movements of these parts of the body."[171]

On the other hand, Spieghel's writings are replete with discussions of other humoral disruptions for which there is no similar protection. For example, "if the heart and lungs become strongly inflamed, an abundance of blood will suddenly rush into the aorta," and this will distend the arteries and produce various functional disorders.[172] Even more dangerous, however, can be the result of some cause such as an unseasonable cold bath, which repels the blood inward:

In the cardiac disease, blood deserts the external parts of the body and rushes to the interior parts, and especially to the heart. This is easily proven by the fact that in such cases the exterior parts are cold, the inner regions are hot, and the pulse becomes worm-like.... Because of the abundance of blood contained in its ventricles, the heart cannot properly carry out its movements of disatole and systole, and so it happens that the patients suffocate and suddenly die, unless they are relieved by bloodletting.[173]

Thus rapid inward movement of the blood can occur, but for Spieghel it had overwhelmingly negative connotations, for not only does this directly deprive the outer parts of the body of their needed warmth, it also paralyzes the very mechanisms by which the balance might otherwise be restored, namely the heartbeat and pulse.

Altogether, then, the range of Spieghel's interests included most, indeed nearly all, of the elements that would enter into Harvey's theory of circulation. Spieghel was, moreover, very much like Harvey in being quite open-minded with regard to most physiological questions, and was rather self-consciously innovative in his ideas about the movement of the heart and blood. And yet, far from emerging with any conception of the circulation, Spieghel remained convinced that underlying all of these diverse phenomena there is a basic, normal pattern of outward movement through both the arteries and the veins.

The Early Harvey

In 1616 William Harvey began teaching anatomy at the London College of Physicians, and by remarkably good fortune the notes which he prepared for these lectures are among the very few of his manuscripts to have survived.[174] They provide us with an invaluable insight into his ideas and interests at a stage when they were already well matured, but before his discovery of the circulation.[175] In retrospect, they seem to reveal a man whose thinking about the movement of the heart and blood was not so different from that of his contemporary Spieghel: he was already deeply immersed in the investigation of this particular subject and quite familiar with most of the basic phenomena that would later enter into his theory of circulation, but was apparently unaware that something like the circulation might remain to be discovered.

From a theoretical point of view, the most distinctive feature of Harvey's anatomical lectures is his affirmation of the notion of the primacy of the blood, which was a marked departure from the traditional view that some formed organ, usually the heart, is the most important component of the organism.[176] For Harvey, the blood's primacy entailed two distinct but related aspects: in embryonic development a drop of blood is the first part to be generated and to live; and within the mature organism the blood is not only a nutritive substance, but also the ultimate repository of heat and spirits, and thus the source of vitality for the rest of the body. Accordingly, throughout his lectures Harvey showed a particular interest in the blood, in its qualities, quantity, distribution, and motion. Following Aristotle, he regarded the presence or absence of red blood as the basic criterion for separating the more from the less perfect animals, and among the blooded animals it is the amount of blood (and hence of heat) that determines the basic differences between species, as well as individual variations within species. Thus both species and individuals among the higher animals are variously described as possessing "more blood," as being "more crammed with blood," as "abounding in a larger quantity of blood," and as "abounding greatly in blood and heat."[177]

Similarly, among the regions and organs of the individual body there are important differences with regard to distribution of blood. Above all, the greatest aggregation of blood occurs with the thorax, and more particularly within the chambers of the heart and the vessels of the lungs. With regard to the auricles and ventricles of the heart, Harvey variously asserted that they are "so filled with blood," are "most crammed with blood," are like "lakes or cysterns of blood," contain "an abundance of blood" or "a multitude of blood," so that the heart is indeed "most stuffed with blood, as is not other viscus."[178] Harvey made it quite clear that it is only in virtue of this contained blood, and not of its own inherent qualities, that the heart may be considered the font of life for the rest of the body.[179] He also described the lungs as "filled" or "crammed with blood," and as possessing "an abundance of blood."[180] Other, lesser concentrations of blood are to be found within the sinuses of the brain, as well as in the liver and spleen.[181]

Statements such as these tend to convey a rather static impression, but

from other passages it is clear that Harvey had a definite notion of a progressive movement of blood through the various parts of the body. Fresh
blood is formed from ingested food, and so the journey begins in the digestive
organs. From there the food is conveyed by the portal veins to the liver, where
(with an important assist from the spleen) the basic conversion to venous
blood is carried out.[182] The blood then passes into the vena cava and its
branches, whose principal function is to supply blood to the right ventricle of
the heart.[183] From there the blood passes through the lungs to the left ventricle, and so on to the arteries.[184]

The basic purpose of the blood's passage through the lungs is to be
tempered through contact with respired air, but in the most perfect animals
the lungs themselves are so crammed with hot blood that the freshly added
venous blood is further concocted into arterial blood, a change which Harvey
regarded as even more important than the earlier formation of venous blood
in the liver.[185] As he put it,

The lungs are the noblest part of the body (with the exception of the heart), insofar as
they are the font of blood. Without the liver you cannot survive for a prolonged period,
but without the lungs not even for a moment. Through the liver passes all the incom-
ing aliment, but through the lungs pass incessantly all the aliment and the whole mass
of the blood, whence the arterial blood is redder. The lungs generate spirit, or rather,
in my opinion, they imbue the aliment [with spirit].[186]

From this statement one might suppose that no blood whatever is absorbed
from the veins prior to the passage through the lungs, but in numerous other
places Harvey indicated that the various parts of the body do indeed receive
blood from the veins as well as from the arteries.[187] Thus the probable meaning of this statement is that in the higher animals, above all in man, the need
for hotter and more spirituous aliment is so great that much the larger part of
the blood from the veins passes through the heart and lungs to the arteries, in
order to acquire this extra perfection.[188]

Harvey also refers here to the consequences of dysfunction of the liver
and lungs, and this typifies a pervasive concern in the lectures not only with
the basic structure and functions of the organs, but with their manifold
variations under a wide range of circumstances. In his section on the skin, for
example, he mentioned the phenomenon of goose-flesh, and gave a typical
Harveian litany of things that can bring it about: "fear, febrile chills, exposure to cold, sleeplessness, disease."[189] Furthermore, such matters are not
only frequently mentioned in passing, but for each organ Harvey routinely included a special survey of pathological changes which he and others had

observed post-mortem.[190] Many of these changes were structural, but Harvey clearly asserted the priority of dietetic and humoral factors in pathological processes: "From errors in diet results cacochimia [general humoral depravity], the persistence of which leads to cachexia [corruption of the solid parts], from which follows corruption of the organs."[191]

Accordingly, Harvey's lectures reveal an intimate familiarity with the categories of humoral pathology, including targeted humoral fluxes, which result in localized problems of excess and defect.[192] As an example of such abnormality, Harvey mentioned an ulcer in the mouth which resulted in excessive salivation, so that "in three days more fluid [was produced] than could be contained in the entire skull."[193] Similarly, the intestines sometimes "abound in humors, or mucous," and thus will benefit from purgation, while the skin is easily discolored by "peccant humors," such as bile in jaundice.[194] However, in keeping with his general outlook Harvey paid particular attention to pathological variations in the distribution of blood. In inflammations, for example, the intestines are found with their "veins large and distended," and with a purplish, blackening color, while in other conditions they are white and livid, "lacking in blood."[195] Concerning the liver Harvey reported, "I have seen it russet, hard, contracted, and lacking in blood," but on the other hand "when inflamed it is distended, blackening, replete with blood."[196] Similarly, in some diseases the spleen is "crammed with blood, like a bag of blood," and he had also observed the veins of the brain to be "distended with blood."[197] And while the auricles of the heart are normally "so filled with blood," Harvey noted that this can especially be seen at autopsy "in those who were strong spirited or subject to anger, or who had suffocated during a fever."[198] Here he probably had in mind the notion of inward concentration of blood that was traditionally associated with such conditions. Finally, Harvey was also familiar with the massive internal haemorrhage, reporting as his own observation that in consequence of a uterine abscess, "all the blood had escaped into the abdominal cavity."[199]

What are the causes of these various movements and aggregations of blood, both in health and disease? No single answer can be given, for the Harvey of 1616 clearly assumed that a diversity of factors is involved. For one thing, he was quite explicit in his adherence to the Galenic theory of natural faculties, according to which every part of the body has the power to attract, retain, and concoct its nutritive humors, as well as to expel its excrements.[200] When all goes well, and the humors "are governed by nature," these processes are entirely beneficial, but when things are "contrary to nature," the excrements wind up in the wrong places, causing disease.[201] As additional factors in the praeternatural movements of the humors Harvey listed the powers of attraction associated with heat, pain, and vacuum, while the simple downward tendency of the humors can also cause certain kinds of swelling.

Harvey also outlined his own theory of spontaneous movements of the humors, according to which every substance that comes under the influence of the innate heat of the body has an inherent tendency to move to a place that is proper for it, analogous to the tendency of each of the four Aristotelian elements to seek its own proper sphere in the Macrocosm.[202] In his lectures Harvey did not explicitly apply this theory to the blood,[203] but from his repeated references to the great abundance of blood within the thorax, it seems reasonable to infer that this is the place to which the blood tends spontaneously to move, all other things being equal. However, this would not have been the only factor promoting the aggregation of blood within the thorax, for according to Harvey the power of attraction depends upon the innate heat, and as the hottest region of the body the thorax would presumably be the most potent in drawing blood to itself.[204] Indeed, if left unopposed this centralized aggregation would effectively deprive the rest of the body of its supply of nourishing and vivifying blood, and it was probably for this reason that Harvey had a very keen interest in mechanical agencies which have the specific effect of propelling blood outward through the body. Thus in listing secondary uses of the respiratory movements he stated with unmistakable emphasis "NB WH perhaps it forces blood and spirits to the intestines and the limbs."[205]

Above all, however, Harvey looked to the heartbeat, and more particularly to the powerful contractions of the heart, as a crucial biological activity whose primary purpose is to continually force blood outward through the arteries to all the parts of the body. His appreciation of the nature and purpose of the movement of the heart was based upon extensive investigations *in vivo*, whose results he summarized in a fairly long section of his anatomical lectures.[206] He brought diverse anatomical and vivisectional data to bear on the issue, but near the end of his discussion he was able to reduce the heartbeat and arterial pulse to three simple principles:

Action [of the heart]: thus relaxed, receives blood
                        contracted, scups it over.
                        In the entire body the arteries respond
                        as my breath in a glove.[207]

Despite its brevity, this summary contains two clear mechanical analogies, that of scupping, which illustrates the role of cardiac contraction in transmitting blood, and that of inflating a glove, which exemplifies the nature of the arterial pulse as a passive mechanical consequence of that transmission. Moreover, this mechanical emphasis is apparent throughout Harvey's discussion of the heartbeat and pulse, which is replete with terms such as "protrude," "impel," "propel," "impulse," "impetus," and "force."

Immediately after giving this summary of the cardiac cycle, Harvey went on to ask the question, "For what purpose?" and his principal suggestion was, "Perhaps the parts are warmed by the arterial blood, which is why, when arteries are obstructed, the parts [supplied by them] become cold."[208] The reference to arterial obstruction again reminds us of his deep-seated medical concerns, and indicates that the heart's propulsion of blood, like all other bodily functions, is subject to disruption or alteration under unusual or pathological circumstances. Indeed, he went on to suggest an additional purpose of the heartbeat having to do entirely with such conditions: "WH perhaps this is of service for the dissipation of heat in fevers, and strong emotions that result from heat."[209] Harvey considered heat to be inseparable from the blood, and this suggestion recalls the observation reported earlier in the lectures that "those who have suffocated during fevers," or who were subject to strong emotions, are found post-mortem to have an unusual amount of blood in their hearts. Thus the point of the suggestion would seem to be that just as blood can sometimes move toward the heart in abnormal amounts, threatening it with an excess, so the heart can to some extent rid itself of the burden by increasing its outward propulsion.

In another passage Harvey pointed to a relationship between the heartbeat and various localized pathological processes, expanding upon the idea that "when arteries are obstructed the parts become cold." This occurred in a summary of his views on the mechanical character of the arterial pulse, under the general heading, "Hence the pulse of the arteries results not from an inherent faculty, but from the heart's protrusion [of blood]."[210] Harvey listed several categories of evidence that had a bearing on this conclusion, including "the experiment with ligatures." In the subsequent expansion of the latter point he stated, "Hence when arteries are obstructed the result is lividity and gangrene," and shortly afterward the two points are brought together in the statement that the propulsive force of the heart is revealed "by the experiment of the ligature, in gangrene."[211] From all of this it seems reasonably certain that by "the experiment with a ligature" Harvey meant the placing of a very tight band around an extremity, which cuts off the influx of arterial blood, and thus eliminates the pulse and makes the part cold. And his further references to lividity and gangrene indicate a relationship between the experimental effect and these pathological conditions, which must also result from the deprivation of blood from the heart.

However, in the same passage Harvey also referred to the opposites of these conditions, namely the distention that results from moderately tight ligation, and inflammation and swelling in general:

Hence from ligatures there is attraction to a part, and thus the reason why, as a result of pain and inflammation, there occurs swelling and the attraction of humors, namely through the arteries.[212]

At first glance it might seem that Harvey was simply affirming the traditional view that moderate ligatures have the power to attract blood, as do heat and pain, and this interpretation could be corroborated by the fact that elsewhere he did affirm the attractive power of the latter two agents. Indeed, his very use of the term "attraction" would seem to leave little room for doubt in this regard.

In fact, though, the terminology is inconclusive, because later in *De motu cordis* Harvey repeatedly used the term "attraction" to describe these same phenomena, while at the same time asserting that their actual cause is the propulsive power of the heart, and not true attraction.[213] And I would suggest that his remarks in the lectures were probably intended to indicate a similar relationship between localized swelling and the heartbeat, rather than simply to reaffirm the traditional views. For why bring up the whole subject under the rubric of "the protruding heart" if not to suggest some such connection? Second, why specify "namely through the arteries" if the focus was indeed on peripheral attraction in the causal sense? Presumably blood could be attracted just as well through the veins, but Harvey does not mention the latter vessels in this passage. Third, a new theory of abnormal swelling based upon the heartbeat would have a direct link with the main physiological issue under discussion, namely the role of the heart in *normally* distending the arterial system every time it contracts, which by simple exaggeration could produce *abnormal* distention "through the arteries." In fact, it was a commonplace among Harvey's predecessors to say that swelling in general, including that under moderate ligation, results from "Nature" sending a rush of blood and spirits, and so the only new elements in such a theory would be to substitute the heartbeat for the indefinite Nature, and to specify the arteries as the channels of the influx.[214]

Thus I would conclude that, in Harvey's view, the normal function of the heart in propelling blood through the arteries was subject both to diminution and to increase under unusual conditions, leading to defect and excess, respectively. Both of these might take the form of spontaneous pathological processes, resulting on the one hand in lividity or gangrene, and on the other in inflammation and swelling. Both might also result from therapeutic intervention, in the form of either tight or moderate ligation. And the same techniques could also be used on an experimental basis to show the effects of cardiac propulsion, both negatively and positively.

Another indication of the potential danger of the heart's contraction is Harvey's repeated assertion that arteries have much thicker walls than veins in order to sustain the impetus of the heartbeat, the clear implication being that without such added protection the arteries would be at risk of physical damage.[215] Moreover, in his longest discussion of this matter Harvey extended it to the issue of why the veins have valves, but the arteries do not:

Hence neither the vena cava nor the pulmonary vein have such a structure [i.e., thick walls like the arteries] because they do not pulsate, but rather are subject to attraction. And this [the absence of pulse in the veins] is because contraposed valves break off the pulse, both in the heart and in other veins. WH hence the reason why the veins have many valves opposed to the heart, but the arteries none, except at their exit from the heart [i.e., the aortic valve], and that set in a contrary manner. Hence the latter vessels [the arteries] are pulsatile, but the former [the veins] are not.[216]

This is an interpretation of the venous valves that is notably different from previous ones, and I would suggest that it is based upon the following reasoning. The principal function of the veins, in Harvey's view, is to supply blood to the heart during its passive diastole, under the relatively gentle influence of the attractive power of the innate heat. The arteries, by contrast, convey blood away from the heart under the violent impact of cardiac systole, hence the greater thickness of their walls. However, so powerful is the heartbeat that it might even propel the venous blood outward, which would not only disrupt the orderly transmission of blood to the arteries, but might also damage the thin-walled veins. Thus to make sure that nothing comparable to outward arterial transmission occurs through the veins, they have been provided with inward-facing valves which "break off" the effect of the heartbeat on their blood.

Harvey undoubtedly formulated this interpretation in conscious opposition to the view of his teacher Fabricius that the venous valves exist chiefly to prevent forceful outward movement due to gravity and peripheral attraction,[217] and the change provides another clear indication of the supreme importance which Harvey attached to the heartbeat among the various factors which might cause the blood to move outward through the body. As we have

seen, in his lectures he did affirm that swelling might result either from gravity or from attraction by heat, but when it came to explaining why the veins
have been provided with structures to inhibit outward movement, such other
factors apparently paled by comparison with the central propulsion by the
heartbeat. However, Harvey clearly assumed that some outward flow does occur through the veins, and so his theory still resembled that of Fabricius to
this extent, that it was concerned with the inhibition of forceful movement,
and presupposed some degree of valvular incompetence to permit the
gradual outward flow due to causes other than the heartbeat.

Finally, in his lectures Harvey pointed to a clear relationship between
the heartbeat and one other abnormal movement of the blood, namely that
observed in arterial haemorrhage. In fact, he made repeated reference to experiments of "wounded arteries," carried out for the precise purpose of
establishing that the contraction of the heart, rather than active arterial
pulsation, is the underlying cause of the forceful expulsion of blood.[218] Thus
in contrast to Galen and other predecessors he probably supposed that
arterial haemorrhage is due solely to the propulsion of blood from the heart,
and not to any direct passage of blood from veins into arteries at the periphery. However, in common with his predecessors he probably would not
have seen any obvious relationship between the rapidity with which the blood
is expelled in haemorrhage, and the rate of cardiac transmission in the intact
body. Indeed, his whole emphasis on the violence and impetus of cardiac
propulsion would lend itself very well to the traditional view of the haemorrhage as a gross acceleration of movement that occurs when a closed system
is unnaturally opened.[219]

Altogether, then, by 1616 Harvey had achieved a fundamental new
understanding of the nature of the heartbeat, and had also assigned it a role
of essential importance in the hierarchy of bodily functions, that of providing
the whole body with a constant supply of nourishing and vivifying blood. This
idea did not involve the rejection of the more traditional notions of the cause
of the movement of the blood, but it did supercede them to a significant
degree. Moreover, Harvey had already begun to extend his new insight into
the realm of abnormal movements of the blood, which played so prominent a
role in traditional medical thought. Most dramatically, perhaps, the heartbeat was identified as the underlying cause of the arterial haemorrhage. It
was also implicated in localized swelling, including that under moderate ligation, while tight ligation and other forms of arterial obstruction were shown
to produce their effects by blocking the passage of arterial blood impelled by
the heart. During conditions such as fever and strong emotions blood could

flow to the heart from veins in unusual amounts, threatening death by suffocation, while the heart itself could respond to such challenges by increasing
its transmission of blood through the lungs, to the arteries. Finally, the existence of inward-facing valves in the veins was also attributed to the propulsive power of the heart, which might otherwise have the wholly
undesirable effect of propelling blood outward through the veins.

With the power of hindsight we can see how all of these developments
would eventually converge in the discovery of the circulation, but I would
emphasize that there was nothing inevitable about Harvey's going on to this
further insight, and that as of 1616 he himself probably had no idea that
something so important remained to be unearthed. After all, his predecessors
had argued endlessly about the nature and timing of the events comprising
the heartbeat and pulse, and he had successfully unravelled that knot. Similarly, each of the additional problems to which he applied the resulting theory also had a prehistory as a more or less self-contained topic of discussion,
and there is no indication that Harvey regarded them as anything more than
so many special questions, each requiring a particular explanation in terms of
his theory of the heartbeat. No doubt these and other similar points would
need further refinement before they could be presented to an audience
beyond the College of Physicians, but I believe that the Harvey of 1616 was
someone who thought that he knew the basic lay of the land with regard to
the movement of the heart and blood. Indeed, as I have tried to show elsewhere, it is probable that even before the discovery of the circulation Harvey
proceeded to write a monograph on the movement of the heart, which at that
time seemed to be a finished piece of investigation.[220]

The Discovery of the Circulation

Of course, Harvey did go on to realize that there is something more than
just the heartbeat underlying these diverse phenomena. Obviously these
earlier interests must have done much to prepare him for this realization,
and any interpretation of the discovery of the circulation which did not see it
as *somehow* emerging from the aggregate of his previously acquired knowledge would be seriously deficient. However, this does not mean that the discovery involved nothing more than the accumulation of particulars, or that
every bit of knowledge which preceded it was of equal importance in bringing
it about. For we have Harvey's own clear and unequivocal testimony, dating
from not long after the discovery, that one factor was of overriding impor-

tance in transforming his outlook. This was his thinking about the enormous abundance of blood transmitted by the heart over a relatively short time, from which it became apparent to him that the same blood must continually return to the heart to be retransmitted.[221]

Apart from the fact that this is Harvey's own direct account of the matter, it seems to me that this emphasis on quantitative reasoning is eminently plausible for other reasons as well. For one thing, it has the virtue of being adequate to the task of explaining what transpired, i.e., of enabling us to understand how Harvey overcame the general problem of indeterminacy that pervaded nearly all of the qualitative evidence of the movement of the blood.[222] Furthermore, a discovery based upon the quantitative aspects of cardiac transmission would fit well into the broader pattern of Harvey's interests, which had long included the general issue of the quantity of the blood, on the one hand, and the role of the heart in transmitting blood, on the other.

In fact, one could say that in 1616 there was already an implicit relationship between the two. In his anatomical lectures one of the major ways in which Harvey expressed his interest in quantity was by repeatedly noting the great abundance of blood that is contained in the auricles and ventricles of the heart.[223] On the other hand, in his discussion of the movement of the heart there are equally vivid descriptions of these same chambers becoming visibly emptied and whiter in color each time they contract.[224] Furthermore, he made it quite clear that because of the heart valves the transmission from auricles to ventricles, and from ventricles to arteries, is irreversible.[225] These assumptions were also implicit in his final, authoritative summary of the action of the heart, "thus relaxed, receives blood, contracted scups it over."[226] And eventually, Harvey was able to formulate an argument for the circulation which required little more than this basic idea as a premise:

The panting of the heart is but the pumping about of the blood, in the expansion receiving, and in the contraction sending it out; and it receives so much at every expansion, that considering the great proportion, and the many beatings of the heart in half an hour, it must of necessity come round about.[227]

However, while in retrospect the discovery of the circulation might appear to be a seemingly obvious logical corollary to Harvey's theory of the heartbeat, there were also some powerful factors which probably would have tended to inhibit this realization on his part. For his early interest in the quantity of the blood was very much of a two-edged sword: there was, on the one hand, the notion of normal abundance, to which I just referred, but there was also the concern with pathological excess as a serious threat to health.[228] Moreover, Harvey had a clear awareness of the potential power of the heartbeat to cause such problems, and so it would have seemed almost beyond question that this function must normally be subject to the strictest teleological controls. That is, if the heartbeat can cause abnormal swelling and inflammation in some part of the body by an excessive impulsion of blood through the arteries, then this presupposes that its ordinary effect is to impel blood in just the right amount.[229] And the same Nature who provided the veins with valves and the arteries with thick tunics to protect them against the force of the heartbeat would not then have subjected the whole body to the obvious risk of an unrestrained impulsion of blood. However, it was precisely this possibility of a constant, systemic excess that Harvey would have had to entertain before he could go on to the further realization that blood must continually return to the heart. This is not to say that it would have been impossible for him to begin to have such suspicions, but only to suggest that it was not the sort of thing that would occur to him in a casual way: he would have had to think about the matter quite deliberately and seriously. However, once he did begin to think about his theory of the heartbeat from this point of view, then for the very same reasons just stated he would immediately have sensed the extreme urgency of the issue, and pursued it through to some definitive resolution.

At all events, Harvey made it quite clear in chapter eight of *De motu cordis* that the consideration of quantity represented a major turning point, both in the structure of the treatise and, more importantly, in the original development of his ideas. The chapter is entitled, "On the abundance of blood passing through the heart from the veins to the arteries, and on the circular movement of the blood," which indicates the overall logical connection that Harvey was about to spell out. He began by stating that perhaps his readers would take in stride what he had previously had to say about the role of the heart in simply transmitting blood,

but now, what remains concerning the amount and abundance of the blood that passes through (although it is highly worthy of consideration)—when I have said these things, they may appear so new and unheard of that I not only fear evil to myself from the hatred of some, but I am afraid lest I have all men for my enemies.

Harvey then proceeded to describe his own original pondering of this matter, choosing rather intense language:

Indeed when I had often and seriously considered with myself, and turned over in my mind at even greater length, ...what great abundance there was:[230] how large, that is, would be the amount of blood transmitted [by the heart], and in how short a time that transmission would occur, I realized that the juice of the [freshly] ingested aliment could not supply [this amount], but that we would have the veins emptied, completely drained, and the arteries, on the other hand, disrupted by the excessive intrusion of blood, unless the blood somehow permeates from the arteries back into the veins, and so returns to the right ventricle of the heart.

I began to ponder whether [the blood] might have a kind of movement, as it were, in a circle, and this I afterward found to be true.[231]

Thus in Harvey's own mind, his fundamental innovation was virtually identical with the consideration of the quantity of the blood.

But what made the issue of quantity appear to be so "highly worthy of consideration" even before Harvey knew where it would lead him? Unfortunately he provides us with no insight in this regard. Conceivably, his attention to this matter could have resulted largely from an internal evolution in his thinking, with his broader interest in the quantitative aspects of blood distribution eventually overcoming the inhibitions against suspecting that cardiac transmission might be excessive. However, it is also possible that Harvey was stimulated by an external influence, because in works published during the 1620s several contemporaries actually touched on the question of the overall amount of blood transmitted by the heart.[232]

The most interesting of these for both chronological and substantive reasons was a physiological treatise *De subtilitate* published in 1621 by the Venetian physician and anatomist Emilio Parigiano.[233] In one of the major sections of this book Parigiano presented a new but highly speculative theory of cardiovascular physiology, according to which the aortic valve is incompetent, so that when the left ventricle of the heart contracts it expels blood into the aorta, and when it dilates it receives back the same blood.[234] Parigiano offered numerous arguments in support of this view, among them the following:

But if the valves in the aorta were an impediment to all return, then, since the heart in systole expels the greater part of its blood into the aorta, and that in scarcely a single moment of time, the aorta would be so continually filled [with blood] that it could receive no more, while the heart as well as the superior arteries would be emptied within a few beats, though experience shows that the upper arteries as well as the lower ones are filled with blood. Thus the arterial blood must necessarily undergo a flux and reflux from the aorta.[235]

Parigiano predicts an imbalance of blood within the arterial system, rather than between veins and arteries, but otherwise the terms of his argument are strikingly similar to Harvey's. Moreover, this argument fits into a broader pattern of quantitative reasoning in Parigiano's book, and some of the other instances actually involve hypothetical calculations similar to those used by Harvey in support of the circulation.[236] And as we shall see, as a premise to these calculations Harvey explicitly stipulated that the heart valves would prevent any direct return from arteries to heart, which was Parigiano's solution to the quantitative problem.

It is thus tempting to envision Harvey reading this passage in Parigiano, recognizing the force of the argument in the light of his own vastly superior understanding of the heartbeat, and so setting out on the quest that brought him to his own alternative conception of return flow. However, while we do know that Harvey eventually read Parigiano's book, and more importantly that he probably read this particular passage,[237] there is no evidence of his having done so prior to the discovery of the circulation, apart from the similarities just mentioned, which are suggestive but not conclusive. Nevertheless, it is at least useful to know that an immediate contemporary of Harvey's was also concerned with the issue of the quantity of blood transmitted by the heart, since this in itself makes it seem less extraordinary for Harvey to have raised this question. And I might add that Parigiano for his part recognized the parallel when he later read Harvey's book.[238]

If Harvey leaves us in the dark as to what launched him on his consideration of quantity, his account does make it clear that much of his interest focused on the problematic implications of a copious transmission. These potential difficulties had to do in part with the physiology of nutrition, which had long provided an important context for Harvey's thinking about the movement of the heart and blood. However, a formal consideration of the quantity of cardiac output suggested that there is in fact a gross disproportion between the two processes, a problem epitomized by Harvey's statement that "the juice of the ingested aliment could not supply" the abundance of blood transmitted by the heart.[239] And an even more distressing problem was "that we would have the veins emptied, completely drained, and the arteries, on the other hand, disrupted by the excessive intrusion of blood," which is to say that the heartbeat threatened nothing less than a major disaster within the terms of humoral pathology.[240]

However, from Harvey's point of view the real problem initially posed by the consideration of quantity would have been the realization that such consequences *ought* to follow from the normal activity of the heart, as he understood it, but obviously they do not—the heart beats unceasingly, and yet for some reason it never succeeds in transmitting all the blood from the veins over to the arteries. Thus much of the urgency of the pondering must have derived from the dilemma that if the amount transmitted were *large*, it would pose grave problems, but if it were *small* it would mean that his theory of diastole and systole was seriously in error. More particularly, it would mean that the perceptible filling and emptying of the heart observed in vivisected animals simply does not correspond to what occurs in the intact body.

Such a reexamination of fundamental assumptions can be inferred from Harvey's historical account in chapter eight, which includes a list of empirical factors from which he derived his impressions of cardiac output:

From experimental vivisections, and from the opening of arteries, and multifaceted inquiries.

Also from the symmetry and magnitude of the ventricles of the heart, and of the vessels entering and leaving them (since Nature, who does nothing without purpose, would not have endowed these vessels with so great a proportional size without purpose).

Also from the harmonious and careful design of the valves and fibers, and from the rest of the structure of the heart, and from many other things besides.

The evidence of quantity derived from vivisection would of course have been the most overt, but the inclusion of the other items clearly implies that it would also be suspect: it might represent a gross distortion of the normal situation. Therefore it had to be reinforced by a scrutiny of the structural details of the heart, which showed that the heart was specifically designed to transmit a great deal of blood (because of the size of its ventricles and orifices),[241] and to do so on an irreversible basis (because of the heart valves).[242]

Reference to the heart valves also points to an even more powerful way of overcoming the problem of vivisectional abnormality, namely the method of hypothetical calculations which Harvey presented in chapter nine.[243] Here he pointed out that on the basis of the valves, it is commonly assumed that the heart irreversibly transmits *some* portion of blood at each beat. However, by calculation it can be shown that even if this amount is not large, the aggregate would still exceed the sum total of blood in the body within a short time—in order to escape the force of the numbers one would have to make the transmission at each beat improbably, indeed vanishingly small.

After presenting these calculations in chapter nine, Harvey then offered seemingly direct empirical corroboration through the opening of arteries, the one specific piece of vivisectional evidence that he included in his list in chapter eight. However, in chapter ten he went on to acknowledge that this source of evidence might in fact be suspect. As he put it:

Granted that when an artery has been cut, and a way has been opened, it happens that the blood is poured out praeternaturally, with an impetus; nevertheless, when the body is intact, and no escape has been provided, and the arteries are filled and in their natural condition—it might not happen that so great an abundance passes through, in so short a space of time, so as to require a return of blood.[244]

Harvey responded to this potential objection by appealing to his theory of cardiac diastole and systole, and more particularly to his hypothetical calculations, which thus provided reassurance that something roughly comparable to the arterial haemorrhage must indeed take place within "the intact body."

Whence this interest in "the opening of arteries?" Harvey had already referred to the procedure in his lectures of 1616, but chiefly as evidence of the impetus of the ejected blood, a point of view which could easily divert attention from the copiousness of the evacuation.[245] However, if we think of the experimental opening of arteries with explicit reference to quantity, we find a clear precedent in the works of Galen, who had repeatedly described such procedures precisely to show the massiveness and rapidity of the expulsion.[246] One reason for doing so was to refute the view of Erasistratus that blood enters the arteries only in consequence of their being opened, while another was to defend Galen's own view of normal peripheral exchanges between arteries and veins through the anastomoses. And in the latter context, Galen specifically called attention to the complete draining of the venous system as a result of the opening of arteries, and this was also noted by Harvey as one of the potential consequences of a copious cardiac transmission.

The similarity was probably no coincidence, for when we turn to Harvey's major discussion of arteriotomy as evidence of quantity in chapter nine, we find that he begins the whole discussion with a direct paraphrase of Galen's account:

This is also made plain by sense, to those who observe the dissection of live animals, that not only when a large artery is opened, but (as Galen confirms for man himself) when any artery, even the smallest, has been cut, in the space of one half hour, *the whole mass of the blood would be exhausted* from the entire body, *from the veins as well as from the arteries.*[247]

The reference to Galen was not just incidental, because the rest of this discussion of arteriotomy reflects a clear preoccupation with the specific terms of Galen's treatment of the matter. For example, Harvey presented a detailed explanation of how the arteries might become exsanguinated postmortem, and suggested that this might have given rise to the ancient doctrine of the empty arteries, which was of course a central issue in Galen's examination of the arterial haemorrhage.

More important, Harvey went to some trouble to refute the main positive conclusion that Galen had drawn from this phenomenon, namely that there is a direct passage of blood from veins into arteries at the periphery. Harvey asserted that "the arteries nowhere receive blood from the veins, except by the transmission that occurs through the heart," and then offered both experimental and experiential evidence that it is impossible to empty the veins through arteriotomy without the involvement of a vigorously beating heart.[248] Thus when he suggested, in chapter eight, that in consequence of the abundance of cardiac transmission, "we would have the veins emptied, completely drained, and the arteries on the other hand, disrupted by the excessive intrusion of blood," he was in effect describing Galen's massive haemorrhage, rerouted through the heart and lungs, and further modified to allow for its occurrence within the intact blood vessels.

Moreover the Galenic context would not only have assisted Harvey in defining the problems resulting from abundant cardiac output, it would also have provided an important lead to the solution as well. For the issue of peripheral exchanges from veins to arteries, *and from arteries back to veins,* was a central focus in Galen's discussions of the arterial haemorrhage, and of course the latter idea was also the key to Harvey's resolution of the quantitative dilemma. And it was probably because of his familiarity with Galen's doctrine of peripheral exchanges[249] that Harvey, in his account in chapter eight, placed such exclusive emphasis on the consideration of quantity as his fundamental innovation, and made no attempt at all to explain how he actually thought of the idea of blood returning from arteries to veins. Thus, when he reached this point in the account, Harvey simply stated that he came to see that the veins would be emptied and the arteries over-filled, *"unless* the blood somehow permeates from the arteries back into the veins,"* as if the possibility of resolving the issue in this way could be taken for granted, as indeed it could have been by any physician who was reasonably familiar with Galen's doctrines on vascular physiology.[250]

Furthermore, while the idea of so much blood making the passage from arteries into veins would have been quite unprecedented as a physiological principle, it would not have been without parallel in the context of pathology and therapy. As we have seen, it had been the view of Erasistratus that as excess blood mounts up within the veins it will eventually spill over into the normally empty arteries, and Galen had agreed that under conditions of plethora there is an abnormally large flow from veins into arteries. Galen had also repeatedly quoted and endorsed the dictum of Erasistratus that "veins which have been evacuated will more readily receive back the blood which has spilled over into the arteries," but had maintained that venesection rather than a starvation diet was the most efficient way to accomplish the desired evacuation. These assumptions were also shared by Harvey's more immediate predecessors and contemporaries, and it was perhaps in recognition of this therapeutic principle that they tended to extend the experimental proof of the anastomoses by noting that it is possible to empty all the blood from the arteries by the opening of veins, as well as the reverse.[251] And in this light, it seems to me that we can strengthen our previous conclusion: not only would a physician well-read in Galen be familiar with the idea of blood passing from arteries into veins, but if faced with a situation in which the veins were being emptied and the arteries over-filled, he would recognize in these the ideal conditions under which an augmented movement of blood from arteries into veins *ought* to occur.

Moreover, Harvey himself invites us to view the notion of a copious passage of blood from arteries into veins in the context of therapeutic reasoning, because when he came to defend this part of his theory in chapters eleven and twelve of *De motu cordis,* he relied largely on evidence drawn from therapeutic venesection.[252] He sought to show that whenever a vein is opened, the evacuation never proceeds from more central into more peripheral veins, but always from heart to arteries, and from arteries into veins, i.e., the pathway which his predecessors had thought to be involved only some of the time. He also noted that such outflow, if allowed to continue, could lead to complete exsanguination no less than the arterial haemorrhage. And by a further application of hypothetical calculations he sought to show that such a copious passage of blood from arteries into veins must happen all the time, independently of the therapeutic intervention.

Thus in asserting in chapter eight that the heart would tend to drain the veins and overfill the arteries unless there were a return of blood from arteries into veins, Harvey was in effect using the familiar terms of humoral medicine, to describe a constant quasi-pathological process caused by the heartbeat that is continually counteracted by a quasi-therapeutic process at the periphery, with the two adding up to the new physiological principle of circulation. In this respect, Harvey's theory parallels Galen's physiological doctrine of mutual exchanges through anastomoses, which was based upon the earlier Erasistratean sequence of pathogenesis and therapy mediated through the anastomoses. The empirical proof for both theories was also based in part upon two overtly abnormal phenomena, namely the haemorrhage, in both its arterial and its venous forms. However, Galen's theory continued to be heavily influenced by its abnormal ancestry, so to speak, in that he and his followers took it for granted that the process of exchange is grossly distorted in one direction or the other when arteries or veins are opened. By contrast, Harvey's theory was founded upon a further normalization of the haemorrhage in its quantitative as well as its qualitative aspects. That is, through thinking about the quantitative implications of his theory of the heartbeat, he came to suspect that even within the intact body the heart must be responsible for something very much like a combination of arterial and venous haemorrhage, which exactly cancel each other out.[253] And once he had formed this suspicion, then the consideration of quantity would have ceased to be the pondering of a puzzling dilemma, and become instead an effort to verify a startling new idea.

As this pattern began to take shape in Harvey's mind, then other phenomena long associated with his theory of the heartbeat would also have begun to appear in a new light. For example, he had by 1616 concluded that the venous valves are all oriented toward the heart and serve the purpose of inhibiting the movement of blood away from it, and this view would naturally merge with and reinforce his nascent conception of return venous flow. In chapter thirteen he directly contrasted his old and his new view, indicating two changes of emphasis: first, the valves not only *retard* outward movement through the veins, they completely *prevent* it, "lest blood move from large veins into smaller ones and so rupture them, or cause varicosities;" and second, the valves not only serve this *negative* function, they *positively* promote the inward flow by easily yielding to it.[254] And Harvey went on to verify these and other points relating to the valves and centripetal venous flow by a brilliant series of experiments, clearly inspired by the demonstration of his teacher Fabricius that blood cannot be forced outward through the valves by streaking.

Harvey also devoted a whole chapter to describing and explaining the effects of tight and moderate ligatures in terms of his theory, and here also there are strong elements of continuity with his earlier remarks in the anatomical lectures.[255] He still regarded the tight ligature as a complete obstruction of the arterial channel, which prevents the heart's normal impulsion of blood into the distal portion of the affected limb. Likewise the swelling under moderate ligation was traced back to the propulsive power of the heart channeled through the arteries. Now, however, by paying attention to the quantity as well as the force of the impelled blood, Harvey was able to show that the normal inflow through the arteries must be matched by an equally normal outflow through the veins. Accordingly, the swelling under moderate ligation is no longer to be regarded as the result of an exaggerated *influx* of blood, but instead it is due to the obstruction of the normal venous *efflux*, with the result that the normal arterial influx simply accumulates below the ligature, and more specifically in the veins. And having proposed this new explanation for swelling under moderate ligation, Harvey extended it to "perhaps every flux" and to swelling and inflammation in general, suggesting that they too might be the result of inhibited efflux rather than abnormal influx.[256]

The Circuit of the Blood

These efforts to verify the component parts of the blood's pathway—from veins to heart, from heart through lungs to arteries, from arteries to veins, from veins back to heart—were of course crucially important to Harvey's case, but his own pervasive concern with the copiousness and rapidity of the blood's movement also provided him with a strong sense of the circulation as a unified process which transcends its individual anatomical components. In *De motu cordis* the term most frequently employed to refer to the discovery in this holistic sense was "the circuit of the blood," but this was not sharply distinguished from the alternative "circular movement of the blood." For example, in chapter fourteen he formally summarized his case with the words, "It is necessary to conclude that the blood in animals is driven in a circuit, with a kind of circular movement." Both conceptions, in turn, had a close relationship to a more descriptive summary employing the language of tonic motion. As Harvey stated at one point, "it will be made clear that [the blood] moves in a circuit from here to there and back again, namely from the center to the extremes and from the extremes back to the center."[257] And he also explained that he did not intend the term "circular movement" in a literal sense, but in the metaphorical sense (for which there was ample precedent) of such a steadily reciprocating process.[258]

In his account of the discovery in chapter eight Harvey indicated that such a synthetic conception of the movement of the blood occurred to him quite early, as a direct consequence of his original consideration of quantity. After relating how the problem of too little blood in the veins and too much in the arteries led him to entertain the possibility of return venous flow, he opened a new paragraph with the dramatic assertion, "I began to ponder *[Coepi egomet mecum cogitare]* whether the blood might have a kind of movement, as it were, in a circle, and this I afterward found to be true.''[259] In other words, even before he had attained certainty as to the factual situation, he was already being guided by a unified conception of what he was attempting to prove. And as he went on to make clear, this conception was heavily indebted to a basic principle of traditional natural philosophy, that of the perfection and preservative character of circular movement. Walter Pagel has explored this aspect of Harvey's thought in great depth, and has shown, moreover, that the principle of circularity had a long prehistory as a *topos* in biological thought, especially in relation to the movement of the heart and that of the blood.[260] And in the present volume, Charles Webster has shown the particular importance of such speculations in Harvey's immediate intellectual community.[261] Thus it is hardly surprising that as Harvey's own preliminary musings took on more coherent form, they should have crystallized around the theme of circular movement, and that this should in turn have enhanced his awareness of the potential importance of his new idea—he had found a concrete process corresponding to what so many others had been speculating about in more general terms.

The related principle of tonic movement also had an ancient pedigree as a commonplace in physiological thought, in the notion of a constant inward and outward movement of the innate heat and spirits of the body. Harvey had long considered these two agencies to be inseparable from the blood, and so he might have seen his theory of circulation as being in some sense a concretization or specification of this general principle as well. In this case, however, the idea had also had a relatively concrete application in the explanation of a wide range of unusual bodily phenomena, which were considered to involve massive movements of the blood inward or outward through the body. Numerous passages in *De motu cordis* show that Harvey saw his theory of circulation as subsuming these older motifs,[262] and given their prevalence in traditional medical thought it would be surprising if this perception were a purely retrospective one. In other words, just as such things as the haemorrhage, and ideas about localized excess and defect, contributed significantly to Harvey's working out of the anatomical pathway of the blood, so also these notions of affections of the whole body probably provided a model, perhaps the most important model, for the more synthetic view.

A passage at the end of chapter fifteen is of particular importance for showing a relationship between the idea of circulation and the old notions of concentration and expansion of the blood. The discussion in this chapter was based upon the traditional idea that the heart is the source of heat, spirits, vitality, and aliment for the rest of the body. Harvey sought to demonstrate that two specific conditions are necessary if the heart is to fulfill this role: First, the heart itself must be able to actively propel an adequate supply of fresh, warm blood to all the parts of the body through the arteries. And second, because the blood quickly loses its vivifying qualities once it has been transmitted to the periphery, it must continually return to the heart through the veins, both to make way for freshly impelled arterial blood, and to provide for its own regeneration at the center of the body.

After expounding the importance of the heart in pathological processes and in the physiology of nutrition, Harvey concluded the discussion by commenting further on why the heart had to be a powerful propulsive organ in order to fulfill its life-giving task:

Furthermore, for this distribution and motion of the blood there was need of impetus and violence; and an impulsor, such as the heart is. This is true in part because the blood, of its own accord, readily concentrates and comes together, as toward its principle, or as part to whole, or as drops of water which have been spread over a table come together to form a mass—something that happens especially quickly from slight causes, such as exposure to cold, fear, febrile chills, and other such causes.[263]

This is a perspective which complements that of the first part of the chapter. There Harvey had argued that if the blood were simply transmitted to the periphery, only to stagnate there, it would block the access of fresh blood. Now he maintains that the tendency of the blood to return inward is in fact so strong that physical violence on the part of the heart is required to counteract it, and under certain circumstances even that is not sufficient to prevent an actual concentration from occurring.

Harvey then went on to suggest that the activity of the whole body is an additional important factor in causing the venous blood to return inward:

This need [for an impulsor of blood] also arises because, by the movement of the limbs, and the compression of the muscles, the blood is squeezed from the capillary veins into the smaller branches, and from there into the larger ones, so that it is more prone to move from the circumference to the center than the contrary, *even if the valves [in the veins] posed no obstacle.* Thus for the blood to leave its principle, and enter narrow and colder places, and move against its spontaneous tendency, it has need both of violence, and an impulsor, such as the heart alone is.[264]

Reference to the valves in the veins suggests that Harvey arrived at this important insight into the effect of muscular contraction on the blood in conscious opposition to the views of Fabricius. The latter, it will be recalled, had

maintained that "violent" bodily exercise would generate heat at the periphery of the body, which would in turn tend to draw the venous blood outward.[265] On the contrary, Harvey asserts, muscular action would have the
direct mechanical effect of driving the venous blood inward. Fabricius had
further noted that "anyone attempting even with some violence *[violentia]* to
impel *[impellere]* the blood downward through the veins, would feel the
resistance and power of the valves."[266] Harvey, by contrast, looks to the
dynamics of centripetal venous flow as the chief factor in resisting centrifugal
flow. And while he no longer sees much danger of anything causing the
venous blood to move outward, he of course envisions a constant, violent impulsion of the blood outward through the arteries.

Thus the net effect of this passage is to portray the circulation as a
dynamic tension between the various factors—both mechanical and vitalistic
—which make the blood move from the circumference to the center, and the
heartbeat which constantly strives to overcome this centralizing tendency.
This is a conception of the circulation which captures much of the substance
as well as the form of the ancient doctrine of tonic (tensional) movement. Or-
dinarily the two movements are kept in balance, but under certain circumstances the inward tendency gains the upper hand, to produce the concentration of blood so familiar in traditional medicine. And although Harvey does
not say so, it seems reasonable to assume that under other conditions an
augmented heartbeat would shift the balance toward outward expansion.

Another passage in *De motu cordis* suggests a connection between the
idea of circulation and a familiar phenomenon that was traditionally thought
to involve an integral sequence of inward and outward movements. This was
the paroxysm of intermittent fever, which was one of a handful of medical
problems to which Harvey applied his theory in chapter sixteen. In his view:

At the beginning of tertian fever the morbific cause makes for the heart, it lingers in
the vicinity of the heart and lungs, and causes the patient to be short of breath and
sluggish, because the vital principle is burdened, and the blood is impacted and
thickened in the lungs, and does not pass through (and I speak as one who has observed this at the dissection of those who have died at the beginning of the
accession). . . . But after the heat has increased, the material has been attenuated, the
ways have been opened, and the transit completed, then the whole body is heated, the
pulse becomes larger and more vehement, and the febrile paroxysm occurs. This is
because the praeternatural heat which has been enkindled within the heart is diffused
from there to the entire body through the arteries, together with the morbific cause;
which is then easily overcome by nature, and dissolved.[267]

Harvey included chapter sixteen for the express purpose of illustrating
the great explanatory power of his new theory, but clearly this interpretation

of the febrile paroxysm stood in a more complex relationship to the circulation than that of a simple *a posteriore* deduction. For one thing, in its broad outlines the account of the paroxysm is not so different from the one given by Galen, and commonly repeated in the textbooks. Harvey has added his distinctive mark by stressing the importance of cardiac transmission, which is first hindered during the inward (cold) stage, then augmented during the outward (hot) stage. However, in his lectures of 1616 he had already pointed to an important role for the heartbeat as a fever-fighting mechanism, along with its more usual function of propelling arterial blood. Indeed, he had even mentioned the post-mortem engorgement of the heart in those who had "suffocated during a fever."[268]

To view Harvey's theory of circulation as a fever made normal through the intervention of quantitative reasoning would be extreme, though it will seem perhaps less so if attention is called to an interesting terminological point: Harvey's favorite term for his discovery was "circuit," and this was a term whose most common medical usage had previously been in reference to the intermittent paroxysm. The term also had, of course, the ordinary meaning of "way around" or "period" and this was probably what Harvey primarily intended by it.[269] However, for an educated physician it probably would not have been possible to speak of a "circuit of the blood" without evoking at least some thought of a regularly recurring disease pattern, notably the malarial paroxysm.[270]

At all events, Harvey made it quite clear that neither the consideration of the quantity of the blood nor the notion of a circuit which it generated could be viewed as strictly physiological issues, in sharp distinction from the processes of disease. After presenting his hypothetical calculations in support of the circulation in chapter nine, he looked forward to the day when he would be able to publish real figures as to the amount of blood transmitted by the heart. He then offered a foretaste of this projected study:

Meanwhile, this I know, and I wish all to be advised of it, that sometimes blood passes through [the heart] in greater abundance, sometimes in less, and so the circuit of the blood is sometimes completed more quickly, and sometimes more slowly, according to temperament, age, external and internal causes, the things natural, and the non-naturals, including sleep, quiet, food, exercise, passions of the soul, and the like.[271]

Thus after having been elevated, so to speak, from the realm of the special effect to that of the constant process, the circulation in its turn became the substrate of great variability under a wide range of circumstances, including ones which were regarded as having great potential to cause disease.

This indicates once again that Harvey never abandoned the point of view according to which physiological and pathological processes are freely continuous with each other, so that it is impossible to say with any certainty where the one leaves off and the other begins. His early investigation of the heartbeat may have constituted a relatively insulated piece of specialized physiological investigation, but otherwise his study of the movement of the blood had to be carried out in the jungle of traditional humoral pathology, where almost nothing could be regarded unequivocally as either normal or abnormal. Once armed with his theory of the heartbeat Harvey went about the business of trying to impose some order on this chaos, but as far as we can tell he initially did so with the intention of providing reasonably consistent explanations for such known phenomena as the venous valves, the effects of ligatures, the haemorrhage, the process of fever, and the cause of swelling, rather than of extracting from them some basic new principle like the circulation. Indeed, the very need for such a covering theory would not have been apparent to a physician like Harvey whose most fundamental medical conviction was that every bodily process, but above all the movement of the blood, is highly variable according to circumstance.

It is for this reason, I believe, that the consideration of quantity was of such crucial importance for the discovery, serving the function that quantification has so often served in the empirical sciences, as a basis for abstracting from diverse and confusing particulars. In other words, the need for a constant recycling of the blood had to be grasped on the rational level before it could be demonstrated experimentally. It is for this reason too that Harvey continued to regard this as the most definitive proof of the circulation, even after he had developed other, seemingly more empirical methods. Some modern readers have regarded these "qualitative proofs" as more convincing than Harvey's hypothetical calculations,[272] but they are so only to someone who is prepared to ligate, cut, or streak vessels on the assumption that the result will have an unequivocal relationship to normal bodily processes. Harvey was of course trying to convince his readers that this was so, but he could not presume such an attitude, and therefore he had to teach them to count as he had done in order to change their outlook on these particular phenomena.

On the other hand, the passage just quoted about the variability of the circulation also reveals a potentially fatal flaw in the quantitative argument: if it is indeed true that "blood sometimes passes through [the heart] in greater abundance, and sometimes in less," then it is impossible to completely rule out the idea that under normal conditions the amount transmitted is so small as not to require a circulation—the transmission of a large amount of blood may itself be a special effect provoked by the conditions of vivisection.[273] We have seen that Harvey himself probably had to come to grips with this problem as a central issue in his pondering of quantity, but the most he could have done was to achieve a degree of relative confidence in this regard, since there would have been no way for him to tell for certain what goes on in the undisturbed depths of the body. Harvey's degree of confidence was no doubt high in view of the time and trouble that he had already invested in working out his theory of the heartbeat. But if he had been unable to conceive of return venous flow as a way out of the quantitative dilemma, or if for some reason he had found this idea to be beyond the realm of acceptability, then the force of the numbers would ultimately have led him to conclude, however reluctantly, that the normal transmission must be very small, and that he had indeed been seriously misled in his understanding of the heartbeat by the distortions of vivisection.

Consequently, while I believe it is true to say that there would have been no theory of circulation without the consideration of quantity, it is equally true that the discovery might never have occurred but for a multiplicity of other factors—empirical, theoretical, philosophical, perhaps even irrational—which made it possible for Harvey to pursue the issue of quantity to this particular conclusion, rather than to some other. And it has also been my contention that many of these "enabling factors," so to speak, were drawn from the very realm of special effects which, from another point of view, could also be so misleading. Some of these had long existed on the borderland between the normal and the abnormal, including: the arterial haemorrhage, which was both a dangerous result of trauma and an experimental technique; the tight ligature, which was equally a therapeutic and an experimental tool; the venous valves, which were thought to achieve a physiological effect by the prevention of pathological movements; the arterio-venous anastomoses, which were originally conceived as a pathogenic mechanism, but later acquired physiological significance as well. Others had existed more exclusively in the realm of the unusual, including the general notions of excess and defect as basic pathogenic mechanisms; the therapeutic tools of moderate ligation and venesection, including the relief of arterial congestion by way of the veins; and the processes of generalized expansion and concentration of the blood, which were thought to occur under a wide variety of conditions, ranging from relatively commonplace emotional events to such serious disease symptoms as the febrile paroxysm. As inherited by Harvey, these complexes of experiential phenomena, of practical techniques, and of theoretical assumptions exemplified to a unique degree the element of uncertainty which pervaded the whole subject of the movement of the blood, but in the light of his theory of the heartbeat and of his consideration of the quantity of the blood, they also provided him with some of the chief building blocks for the broader theory of circulation.

It might seem paradoxical that the medical context should have played this dual role, but it is difficult to see how it could have been otherwise. For it was simply the case that at Harvey's time the richest body of experiential and theoretical knowledge about the movement of the blood lay in the areas of pathology and therapeutics, so that if he were going to think about the question at all he had necessarily to concern himself with these subjects. And if he thought about them, he necessarily laid himself open to being influenced both positively and negatively by the existing assumptions that he found there.

However, it has not been my intention in this essay either to praise or to blame the medical context of Harvey's discovery, nor to try to say on balance whether its positive effects outweighed the negative. Rather, I have tried simply to show the inescapable relevance of this context for understanding the achievement of someone who was, after all, not only an Aristotelian natural philosopher and a devotee of anatomical research, but a medical practitioner as well, reared in the Hippocratic and Galenic tradition of humoral pathology, and faced with problems of disease and therapy on a daily basis.

Notes

1. This section has benefited from the suggestions and criticisms of Dr. Owsei Temkin, though I am of course solely responsible for the final result.
2. On dietetic medicine in general, see Ludwig Edelstein, "The Dietetics of Antiquity," in O. and C. L. Temkin, eds., *Ancient Medicine. Selected Papers of Ludwig Edelstein* (Baltimore: Johns Hopkins, 1967), pp. 303-16. On the relationship between dietetics and medical theory, see O. Temkin, "Der systematische Zusammenhang im Corpus Hippocraticum," *Kyklos,* 1928, *1:* 9-43, esp. pp. 34-36; idem, "Greek Medicine as Science and Craft," in his *The Double Face of Janus and Other Essays in the History of Medicine* (Baltimore: Johns Hopkins, 1977), pp. 137-53, esp. 147-53; and idem, *Galenism, Rise and Decline of a Medical Philosophy* (Ithaca, N.Y.: Cornell University Press, 1973) esp. pp. 38-42, and 153-56.
3. On the background and long survival of this three-fold division, see L. J. Rather, "The 'six things non-natural': a note on the origins and fate of a doctrine and a phrase," *Clio Medica,* 1968, *3:* 337-47; Saul Jarcho, "Galen's six non-naturals: a bibliographic note and translation," *Bull. Hist. Med.,* 1970, *44:* 372-77; J. Bylebyl, "Galen on the non-natural causes of variation in the pulse," *Bull. Hist. Med.,* 1971, *45:* 482-85; Peter H. Niebyl, "The non-naturals," *Bull. Hist. Med.,* 1971, *45:* 486-92.
4. See, e.g. Jean Fernel, *Physiologia,* esp. ii, preface, in *Opera medicinalia* (Venice, 1566), p. 69.

5. See refs. in note 3 above.

6. Temkin, *Galenism*, pp. 17-18, 102.

7. See, e.g., Fernel, *Pathologia*, esp. i. 1, 2; *Opera*, pp. 219-21.

8. Max Neuberger, *Die Lehre von der Heilkraft der Natur im Wandel der Zeiten* (Stuttgart: Enke, 1926), pp. 5-58.

9. Such a conception of the human body as a corollary to dietetic medicine is well described by Edelstein, "Dietetics," pp. 303-4.

10. For a good illustration of this attitude, see Hippocrates, *On the Nature of Man*, ed. and tr. W. H. S. Jones (Loeb Classical Library), IV, 2-41.

11. For an analysis of related issues in medical thought of the nineteenth century, see G. Canguilhem, *Le normal et le pathologique*, 2nd ed. (Paris: Presses Universitaires de France, 1972), esp. part I. I am grateful to Drs. Ruth Fried and William Coleman for bringing Canguilhem's essay to my attention.

12. Compare, for example, the differing views of Galen and Erasistratus regarding inflammation and its relation to normal processes, pp. 39 and 47 below.

13. See Temkin, "Der systematische Zusammenhang," passim.

14. See, for example, Hippocrates, *On the Nature of Man*, 4-6; ed. and tr. Jones, IV, 11-19, and compare with Galen, *On the Natural Faculties*, ii. 9; ed. and tr. A. J. Brock (Loeb Classical Library), pp. 205-17.

15. Edelstein, "The History of Anatomy in Antiquity," and "The Relation of Ancient Philosophy to Medicine," in *Ancient Medicine*, pp. 247-301, and 349-66; Temkin, *Galenism*, pp. 41-42, 65-66.

16. See Galen *De locis affectis* iii and iv, passim, for many such insights; in *Claudii Galeni Opera omnia*, ed. C. G. Kühn, 20 vols. (Leipzig, 1821-33), VIII, 135-296. Subsequent references to this edition will be to 'K' and the volume number.

17. Edelstein, "Anatomy in Antiquity," pp. 269-70; and "Ancient Philosophy and Medicine," pp. 351-53.

18. Temkin, *Galenism*, pp. 18, 28-35.

19. Aristotle, *History of Animals*, e.g. i. 17 and iii. 2; ed. and tr. A. L. Peck (Loeb Classical Library), I, 65, 67, 163.

20. Celsus *De medicina* Proem. 40-44; ed. and tr. W. G. Spencer (Loeb Classical Library), I, 23-25.

21. *Ibid.*, 23-26, 40-44; tr. Spencer, pp. 15, 23-25. See also Lloyd G. Stevenson, "Anatomical Reasoning in Physiological Thought," in C. McC. Brooks and P. F. Cranefield, eds., *The Historical Development of Physiological Thought* (New York: Hafner, 1959), pp. 27-38, esp. pp. 29-30.

22. The classic instance of this in antiquity occurred in the dispute on blood in the arteries, discussed below, pp. 46-51. Objections based on vivisectional distortion were frequently raised by early critics of the theory of circulation. See, e.g., Nikolaus Mani, "Jean Riolan II (1580-1657) and medical research," *Bull. Hist. Med.*, 1968, *42:* 128, 130-31, 139-44. For the persistence of this attitude toward vivisection see e.g., Stevenson, "Anatomical Reasoning," pp. 34-36, and Canguilhem, *Le normal*, p. 21.

23. See below, pp. 44-45, 49-51, 61, 63, 69-72, 82-83.

24. Such appeals to medical experience are especially frequent in Harvey's case for the circulation in chapters 9-16. See *Exercitatio anatomica de motu cordis et sanguinis in animalibus* (Frankfurt, 1628), pp. 45-64, passim. (Henceforth cited as *DMC*). See also the remarkable sequence of experimental and pathological observations in *Exercitationes duae anatomicae de circulatione sanguinis ad Joannem Riolanum*, Ex.II; in Harvey, *Opera omnia: a collegio medicorum Londinensi edita* (London, 1766), pp. 125-29.

25. E.g., *DMC* ch. 10, pp. 47-48; and ch. 13, p. 58.

26. Ibid., ch. 9, pp. 45–46; and Proem, p. 14.

27. *Iliad* xiii. 442–44; and xvi. 481; ed. and tr. A. T. Murray (Loeb Classical Library), II, 35, 201.

28. F. R. Hurlbutt, Jr., *"Peri kardies.* A treatise on the heart from the Hippocratic Corpus: introduction and translation," *Bull. Hist. Med.,* 1939, *7:* 1111 (translation slightly altered).

29. Galen, *On Anatomical Procedures,* vii. 12; tr. Charles Singer (London: Oxford University Press, 1956), pp. 190–97.

30. Vesalius, *De humani corporis fabrica libri septem* (Basel, 1543), pp. 660–63.

31. *DMC* ch. 10, p. 47.

32. J. J. Bylebyl, "The growth of Harvey's *De motu cordis,"* *Bull. Hist. Med.,* 1973, *43:* 434–38.

33. Ibid., pp. 429–33.

34. *DMC,* Proem, p. 10.

35. I have discussed these aspects of the discovery in "The growth of *DMC,"* pp. 428–40, and "Nutrition, quantification, and circulation," *Bull. Hist. Med.,* 1977, *51:* 369–85.

36. Harvey, *Prelectiones anatomiae universalis,* p. 80v (for full reference, see note 174 below).

37. Temkin, *Galenism,* p. 158, note 57.

38. Temkin, "Systematische Zusammenhang," pp. 14–23.

39. On the commonness of the notion of "flux" in early Greek medical thought, see Temkin, "Greek Medicine as Science," p. 146.

40. *Des Hémorrhoïdes,* 1; in *Oeuvres complètes d'Hippocrate,* ed. and tr. E. Littré, 10 vols. (Paris: 1839–61), VI, 436–37.

41. For ideas about wounds and their treatment, see the treatise *On Ulcers,* in *The Genuine Works of Hippocrates,* tr. Francis Adams, 2 vols. (New York: Wood, 1886), II, 293–306, esp. pp. 295, 305–6. Cf. also *Nature of Man,* 6; tr. Jones, IV, 15–19, where the flow of blood following a wound is compared to the action of purgative drugs on the other humors. See also Peter H. Niebyl, "Venesection and the Concept of the Foreign Body: A Historical Study in the Therapeutic Consequences of Humoral and Traumatic Concepts of Disease" (Ph.D. dissertation, Yale University, 1969), pp. 38–46; and Guido Majno, *The Healing Hand. Man and Wound in the Ancient World* (Cambridge, Mass.: Harvard University Press, 1975), pp. 150–200.

42. *On Ulcers,* 14; tr. Adams, p. 305.

43. Hippocrates, *Aphorisms,* vii. 54; tr. Jones, IV, 205–7.

44. Hippocrates, *Nature of Man,* 11; tr. Jones, IV, 33. For a general discussion of Hippocratic bloodletting, see Niebyl, "Venesection," pp. 26–57.

45. Ibid., p. 43.

46. *Epidemics* ii. 3. 14; ed. Littré, V, 116.

47. H. Diels, *Die Fragmente der Vorsokratiker,* 2 vols. (3rd ed.; Berlin, 1912), I, 134, #18.

48. *The Sacred Disease,* 18; tr. Jones, II, 177.

49. *Breaths,* 8; tr. Jones, II, 237.

50. *Regimen,* ii. 64; tr. Jones, IV, 363–65.

51. Ibid., p. 365.

52. Temkin, "Systematische Zusammenhang," p. 30. See also *Nature of Man,* 11 and *Regimen in Health,* 7; tr. Jones, IV, 33, 55; *Des chairs,* 13; tr. Littré, VIII, 601.

53. Galen, *On the Natural Faculties,* ed. and tr. Brock, passim.

54. See, e.g., *De differentiis febrium* ii. 13; K 7, 381–82. Cf. also *Nat. facs.* i. 11, tr. Brock, p. 41; and iii. 12, p. 287: "In all organs, then, both their natural effects and their disorders and maladies plainly take place on analogous lines."

55. *De sanitate tuenda* iv. 11 and vi. 6; K 6, 300–303, 407–10.

56. *Nat. facs.* iii. 13; tr. Brock, pp. 295–97.

57. *De diff. feb.* ii. 5, 11; K 7, 345, 374–75; *Ad Glauconem de medendi methodo* ii. 1; K 11, 71–78. See also Niebyl, "Venesection," pp. 129–30.

58. *De diff. feb.* ii. 15; K 7, 384-6; *Methodus medendi* xiii. 3; K 10, 877-79.

59. On the relationship between localism and generalism in Galenic pathology, see Niebyl, "Venesection," pp. 96-142, passim.

60. *De diff. feb.* ii. 14; K 7, 382-83.

61. Ibid., ii. 17; K 7, 398-99. Galen goes on to note that the same local inflammation can in turn give rise to generalized fever.

62. S. Sambursky, *Physics of the Stoics* (New York: Macmillan, 1959), pp. 21-48.

63. Philo Judaeus, *The Unchangeableness of God.* vii. 35-36; ed. and tr. F. H. Colsen (Loeb Classical Library), III, 27-29. This is Fragment #458 in J. von Arnim, ed., *Stoicorum veterum fragmenta.* 4 vols. (Leipzig: Teubner, 1921-24), II, 149. See also Frs. #442, 447, 448, 451, 454, 802.

64. Ibid., #766-8, 875, 877, 886, 899.

65. *De tremore, palpitatione, convulsione et rigore* 6; K 7, 616-17. Von Arnim, *Stoic. Vet. Frag.* II, 147, #446, regards this passage as reflecting Stoic doctrine.

66. *De tremore,* K 7, 618-26. This statement applies only to the specific notion of inward and outward movement, and not to the more general concept of *tonos.* See O. Temkin, "The Classical Roots of Glisson's Doctrine of Irritation," in *The Double Face of Janus,* pp. 303, 314.

67. *De symptomatum causis* ii. 5; K 7, 191. For the further elaboration of this point, and examples, see pp. 190-96, and also *De sanitate tuenda* ii. 9; K 6, 137-38. See also T. S. Hall, "Greek medical and philosophical interpretations of fear," *Bull. N. Y. Acad. Med.,* 1974, *50:* 825-29.

68. *De plenitudine* 6, 11; K 7, 538-39, 581; *De causis morborum* i. 2; K 7, 4.

69. *De sympt. caus.* ii. 5; K 7, 193-94. See also *De praesagitione ex pulsibus* iii. 7; K 9, 374-75.

70. *Ad Glauc.* i. 2; K 11, 13-14.

71. *De diff. feb.* ii. 3-5; K 7, 339-45. See also chs. 11-18 on the further causal factors in intermittent fevers.

72. *De tremore* 7; K 7, 632-35.

73. Ibid., pp. 633-34. See also *De praesag. puls.* iii. 7; K 9, 374-75, 383-85.

74. *De tremore,* K 7, 634, See also *Commentarius in Hippocrates de acutorum morborum victu* i. 45; K 15, 511-12.

75. *De sanitate tuenda* vi. 8; tr. R. M. Green as *Galen's Hygiene* (Springfield, Ill.: Thomas, 1951), p. 257. See also Galen's "Advice for an epileptic boy," tr. O. Temkin, *Bull. Hist. Med.,* 1934, *2:* 183.

76. *In Hippocratis de medici officina commentarius* iii. 33; K 18b, 892-94.

77. *Methodus medendi* v. 3; K 10, 315-17. See also *On the Medical Sects for Beginners,* 3; tr. A. J. Brock in *Greek Medicine* (London and New York: Dent and Dutton, 1929), p. 135.

78. *De locis affectis* i. 1; K 8, 5; *On Anatomical Procedures,* iii. 1; tr. Singer, p. 61. See also Majno, *The Healing Hand,* pp. 418-20, and below, pp. 49-51.

79. *Methodus medendi* v. 3; K 10, 315-17.

80. For an analysis of Galen's use of bloodletting, see Niebyl, "Venesection," pp. 96-142.

81. *On the Medical Sects,* 3; tr. Brock, pp. 135-36.

82. *Comm. in Hippoc. de acut. morb. vict.* ii. 10; K 15, 533-34.

83. Ibid. See also e.g., *De tremore,* 5; K 7, 603-4.

84. *Commentarius in Hippocrates Epidemiorum II* iii. 24; K 17a, 434-35.

85. *Methodus medendi* v. 3; K 10, 316-17.

86. *In Hipp. de med. offic. comm.* iii. 33; K 18b, 896-909. Cf. also *De locis affectis* iii. 11; K 8, 197-98.

87. *Anat. Proc.* iii. 9; tr. Singer, p. 82; *Methodus medendi* xiii. 22; K 10, 941-42. (The latter passage was pointed out to me by O. Temkin.) See also Majno, *The Healing Hand,* pp. 328, 403.

88. *De usu pulsuum* 3; K 5, 160. In *Anat. Proc.* vii. 12, tr. Singer, p. 193. Galen points out that arterial ligation can lead to gangrene.

89. *De usu puls.* 3; K 5, 160. Earlier in this work (1, p. 150), Galen had noted that when limbs have their arteries ligated, "temporis decursu torpidi, frigidi, pallidi et tabidi evadant." Cf. Harvey, *DMC,* Proem, p. 12: "(si ligaveris arterias) statim partes non modo torpent, frigent, & quasi pallidae cernuntur, sed & ali tandem desinunt, quod secundum Galenum contingit...."

90. *De usu puls.* 1; K 5, 149-50.

91. *Anat. Proc.* vii. 16; tr. Singer, pp. 197-99.

92. *Ibid.* viii. 4-9; pp. 208-22.

93. *De Hippocratis et Platonis Placitis* vi. 3; K 5, 519-21.

94. Compare Galen's neurological experiments (note 92 above) with his descriptions of neuropathology in *De locis affectis* iii and iv, esp. iii. 4 and iv. 5-7; K 8, 208-14, 235-61.

95. *De venarum arteriarumque dissectione* 3; K 2, 790.

96. *Anat. Proc.* iii. 5; tr. Singer, p. 76, slightly modified. Cf. Harvey, *DMC,* ch. 11, p. 49: "Now let an experiment be made on the arm of a man, either by the application of a ligature such as is used in bloodletting or by firmly grasping it with the hand itself. This can be done more conveniently in a thin subject, who has large veins, and when (after the body has been heated), the outer parts are hot, and there is a greater quantity of blood in the extremities."

97. *An in arteriis natura sanguis contineatur* 1; K 4, 703-6.

98. Ibid. 1-5, passim; W. H. S. Jones, ed. and tr., *The Medical Writings of Anonymus Londinensis* (Cambridge: University Press, 1947), pp. 103-9.

99. For a summary of Erasistratus's main doctrines, see J. F. Dobson, "Erasistratus," *Proc. Roy. Soc. Med.,* Feb. 16, 1927, *Sect. Hist. Med.,* pp. 825-32.

100. Jones, *Anonymus Londinensis,* pp. 85-89, 99, 103, 127.

101. Galen, *Nat. Facs.* ii. 1, 6; tr. Brock, p. 117-19, 149-55, 161-65.

102. Dobson, "Erasistratus," pp. 828-29.

103. Ibid., p. 830.

104. Galen *De plenitudine* 6, 7; K 7, 537-38, 541-42; idem *De venae sectione adversus Erasistratum* 3; K 11, 153-54; H. Diels, ed., *Doxographi Graeci* (Berlin, 1879), p. 441; Celsus *De medicina* Proem. 15, 60; ed. and tr. Spencer, I, 9-11, 33.

105. *De venae sect. adv. Erasist.* 3; K 11, 154.

106. Galen, "On Phlebotomy against the Erasistrateans at Rome," 1, 7; ed. and tr. Ronald F. Kotrc (Ph.D. dissertation, University of Washington, 1970), pp. 178, 210-14.

107. Ibid., 8, pp. 215-17; *De venae sect. adv. Erasist.* 3, 8; K 11, 155-56, 176-79. See also Majno, *The Healing Hand,* p. 335.

108. *Nat. Facs.* passim, esp. ii. 1, 6; and iii. 13, 14; tr. Brock, pp. 117-19, 149-55, 161-65, 313-19; *An sanguis* 6-8; K 4, 725-36; *De usu puls.* passim, esp. 4; K 5, p. 164.

109. *An sanguis* 6-8; K 4, 725-27, 730-32, 734; *De usu puls.* 5; K 5, 168.

110. *An sanguis* 6; K 4, 723-24. But see also *Anat. Proc.,* vii. 16; tr. Singer, pp. 197-98.

111. *An sanguis* 1, 2, 4, 5; K 4, 703-9, 712-18.

112. Ibid. 4; p. 714.

113. Ibid. 2; pp. 706-9.

114. *De usu puls.* 5; K 5, 164-67; *Nat. Facs.,* iii. 13-15; tr. Brock, pp. 313-21.

115. Galen, *On the Usefulness of the Parts of the Body,* vi. 17; tr. M. T. May, 2 vols. (Ithaca, N.Y.: Cornell University Press, 1968) I, 321-24.

116. *De plenitudine* 11; K 7, 573; see also *De causis pulsuum* ii. 2; K 9, 63-65.

117. *On Phlebotomy,* 1, 7; tr. Kotrc, pp. 178, 210-14; *De venae sect. adv. Erasist.* 8; K 11, 176-79.

118. *De usu puls.,* 5; K 5, 165; see also *Nat. Facs.* iii. 15; tr. Brock, p. 321.

119. Caimo, *De calido innato libri tres* (Venice, 1626), p. 178. See also, e.g., Donato Antonio Altomare, *Omnia, quae hucusque in lucem prodierunt, Opera* (Lyons, 1565), pp. 20-21.
120. *De calido,* pp. 179-92. However, Caimo went on (pp. 193-201) to relate the inward and outward movement of the innate heat to the diastole and systole of the heart.
121. Giovanni Argenterio, *De somno et vigilia libri duo* (Florence, 1556), passim, esp. pp. 86-87, 107. Argenterio explicitly related this thesis to Galen's doctrine of inward and outward movement of the innate heat (e.g., pp. 62-63, citing the passage quoted above, note 65).
122. Ibid., pp. 50-53, 56, 64-67.
123. Ibid., p. 87.
124. Ibid.
125. Ibid., p. 63.
126. Ibid., p. 68.
127. Ibid., p. 70.
128. Albertini, *De affectionibus cordis libri tres* (Venice, 1618), p. 227. Quite similar ideas occur in Eustachio Rudio, *De virtutibus et viciis cordis libri tres* (Venice, 1587), e.g., pp. 50r-59v.
129. Albertini, *De affect.,* p. 234.
130. Ibid., p. 387.
131. Ibid., p. 326.
132. Sassonia, *De febribus tractatus* (Venice, 1620), p. 42.
133. See, e.g., Celsus *De medicina* iii. 12.1.; ed. Spencer, I, 12: "febres...quae certum habent circuitum."; Pietro d'Abano, *Conciliator controversiarum, quae inter philosophos et medicos versantur,* Diff. 88, "An humores possint confluere periodice"; (Venice, 1548), fols. 137r-39r; e.g. (137v) "Causa propter quam circuitus febres habent." Galen had written a treatise whose title was translated *Ad eos qui de typis scripserunt vel de circuitibus. (Opera,* [Venice, 1550-51], II, 91v-94v.)
134. Sassonia, *De febribus,* pp. 50-51.
135. G. T. Minadoi, *Disputationes duae, 1. De causa periodicationum in febribus. 2. De febre ex sanguinis putredine* (Padua, 1599), pp. 13-14.
136. Harvey, summarizing the argument of *DMC* in his Letter to Caspar Hofmann. (E. V. Ferrario, F. N. L. Poynter and K. J. Franklin, "William Harvey's debate with Caspar Hofmann on the circulation of the blood. New documentary evidence," *J. Hist. Med.,* 1960, *15:* 14.) Cf. *DMC* ch. 14, p. 58.
137. *De affect.,* p. 387; see also pp. 365, 7.
138. Sassonia, *Prognoseon practicarum libri duo* (Frankfurt, 1610), pp. 194-96. See also Rudio, *De virtutibus,* pp. 53r, 59v.
139. J. B. de C. M. Saunders and C. D. O'Malley, intro. to *Andreas Vesalius Bruxellensis: the Bloodletting Letter of 1539* (New York: Schuman, n.d.), pp. 5-19.
140. Vesalius, *Epistola, docens venam axillarem dextri cubiti in dolore laterali secandam* (Basel, 1539), reprinted in *Opuscula selecta neerlandicorum de arte medica* VIII, 1930, Plate 1, and pp. 44-48.
141. Ibid., p. 22.
142. See, e.g., Francisco de Valles, *Controversiarum medicarum & philosophicarum* (Compluti, 1564) vii. 3, fols. 140v-42r, "De modo quo fluit sanguis in venae scissione," where various views are examined; Laurent Joubert, *Paradoxorum decas prima atque altera* (Lyons, 1566) i. 9, pp. 256-66.
143. E.g., Valles, *Controvers.,* p. 142r: "hinc trahentibus frictione, ligamine & calida;" Joubert, *Paradox.,* p. 257.
144. Leone, *Novum opus quaestionum, seu problematum* (Venice, 1523), problem 74, not paginated.
145. Guidi, *Ars medicinalis,* 3 vols. (Venice, 1611), III, Surgery, pp. 28-29.

146. Joubert, *Paradox.* ii. 8, p. 491.
147. Ibid., i. 10, p. 280.
148. Joubert, *Operum Latinorum tomus primus* (Frankfurt, 1599), p. 112. Sassonia, *Prognoseon,* p. 177; Santorio, *Commentaria in primam fen primi libri canonis Avicennae* (Venice, 1626), cols. 291-92.
149. Platter, *Praxeos medicae tomi tres* (Basel, 1625), I, col. 475. See also Andrea Cesalpino, *Quaestionum medicarum libri II,* published with *Quaestionum peripateticarum lib. V,* 2d ed. (Venice, 1593), p. 212r: "Venas cum arteriis adeo copulari osculis, ut vena secta prima exeat sanguis venalis nigrior, deinde succedat arterialis flavior, ut plerumque contingit."
150. Joubert, *Operum,* p. 112.
151. Ibid.
152. Cesalpino, *Quaest. med.,* p. 234r; cf. also pp. 229r-30r. For a fuller analysis of this whole passage, see Walter Pagel, *William Harvey's Biological Ideas* (New York: Hafner, 1967), pp. 171-78, and also his *New Light on William Harvey* (Basel: Karger, 1976), pp. 39-41.
153. *Quaest. med.,* p. 234r: "Forte recurrit eo tempore sanguis ad principium, ne intercisus extinguatur."
154. Ibid., p. 233v: "Occlusis enim in collo venis, cum sanguis & spiritus permeare nequeunt sursum,...."; *Katoptron, sive speculum artis medicae Hippocraticum* (Frankfurt, 1605), vii. 1, p. 488: "Vena autem cava ramos in totum corpus dispergit, ut simul cum arteriis universas partes nutriant." In addition, the veins have an important, and normal, centripetal function in supplying blood to the heart—see e.g., vi. 19, p. 473: "Continuus quidam motus fieret ex venis in cor, & ex corde in arterias." However, it does not appear that in this context Cesalpino conceived of the veins as *returning* blood to the heart—it is rather a matter of supplying the heart with fresh blood from the liver. (See p. 472, "Vena cava materiam subministrat ex hepate.")
155. *Quaest. med.,* pp. 233v, 234v.
156. Fabricius, *De venarum ostiolis* (Padua, 1603). Facsimile ed. with intro., tr., and notes by K. J. Franklin (Springfield, Ill.: Thomas, 1933), pp. 48-49. T. H. Huxley has pointed out that "The only conclusion which is warranted by the presence of valves in the veins is, that such valves will tend to place a certain amount of obstacle in the way of a liquid flowing in a direction opposite to that in which the valves are inclined." ("William Harvey," *Fortnightly Review,* n.s., 1878, *23:* 187.) This is what Fabricius thought.
157. *De ven. ost.,* p. 48.
158. Ibid., p. 47, my italics.
159. Ibid., translation modified.
160. Ibid., p. 50, translation modified. In his work on praeternatural swelling, Fabricius's teacher Fallopio (*Opera quae adhuc extant omnia* [Frankfurt, 1584], p. 703) had included strong exercise as one cause of this condition: "quando natura vi sua massa sanguinis aliquid transmittat ad partem vel partes, quod patet in valde exercitatus, in quibus massa funditur."
161. Fabricius, *De ven. ost.,* p. 52, translation slightly modified, my italics. Here the streaking procedure is even more closely linked with spontaneous pathological conditions.
162. Ibid., p. 72.
163. Huxley, "William Harvey," p. 179, briefly makes such a comparison. For biographical data, see the article "Spiegel" by G. A. Lindeboom in *Dictionary of Scientific Biography,* vol. XII (New York: Scribner's, 1975), pp. 577-78.
164. Spieghel, *De formato foetu* (Padua, 1626); *De humani corporis fabrica libri decem* (Venice, 1627).
165. Spieghel, *Fabrica,* pp. 150-53, 177-79, 185-86.
166. Ibid., p. 300. See also pp. 187, 199-200, 296, 299.
167. Ibid., p. 187.
168. Ibid., p. 154.

169. Ibid., p. 187. See also pp. 154, 170, 171, 188.

170. Ibid., p. 171: "Secta ergo hac vena, quia proximae anastomoses sunt, fieri nequit, quin sanguis arteriosus quoque effundatur, id quod in cubiti venis incisis non ita fieri potest, ubi anastomoses paulo remotiores a loco in qua vena aperitur."

171. Ibid., pp. 152-53.

172. Ibid., p. 193. See also p. 197.

173. Spieghel, Letter to Gulielmo Sohiero at Venice, n.d., printed in *De form. foet.*, p. 64; cf. *Fabrica*, p. 189. See also p. 300, on the role of the heart in resisting such occurrences.

174. In preparing this account I have relied on both *Prelectiones anatomiae universalis by William Harvey*, ed., with facsimile reproduction, by a committee of the Royal College of Physicians of London (London: Churchill, 1886), and the *Anatomical Lectures of William Harvey. Prelectiones Anatomie Universalis. De Musculis*, ed. with intro., tr., and notes, by Gweneth Whitteridge (Edinburgh and London: E. & S. Livingstone, 1964). Whitteridge's readings are generally superior to those in the 1886 transcript, but the latter has the virtue of preserving the exact format of the notes, which conveys a good deal of meaning in itself. References will be to *PAU* and the page number of the original MS, which is provided in both editions.

175. For earlier analyses of the lectures, see Whitteridge, intro. to *PAU*. pp. xxv-lxiv; G. Keynes, *The Life of William Harvey* (Oxford: Clarendon, 1966), pp. 84-111; Pagel, *Harvey's Biological Ideas*. pp. 209-29; and Whitteridge, *William Harvey and the Circulation of the Blood* (New York: American Elsevier, 1971), pp. 89-103.

176. Different aspects of this idea are discussed or mentioned in *PAU*. pp. 33r, 35, 37v, 38r, 61v, 62r, 72r-75v, 76v, 81r-83v, 85r-87r, 90v, 91r, 92r, 94v. See also Pagel, *Harvey's Biological Ideas*. pp. 222-23. In the immediate aftermath of the discovery of the circulation, which showed that blood must continually return to the heart, Harvey temporarily reverted to the more traditional primacy of the heart, but by the time of his later works he had reconciled the discovery with his older ideas about the blood. See J. Bylebyl, "William Harvey," in *Dictionary of Scientific Biography*. vol. VI (New York: Scribner's, 1972), pp. 157-58.

177. *PAU*. pp. 61v, 62r, 81r-83v, 86v.

178. Ibid., pp. 73r, 74v, 75, 76v, 81r.

179. Ibid., pp. 73r-76v.

180. Ibid., pp. 43r, 81v, 82r, 83r, 86r.

181. Ibid., pp. 38v, 90r, See also 45v.

182. Ibid., esp. pp. 21r, 23v-24v, and 26r-38r, passim.

183. See esp. ibid., p. 74r, where Harvey makes a distinction between the veins "as pathway *(ut via)*" which leads out from the liver, and "as container and reservoir *(ut vas et receptaculum)*" which subserves the heart. He clearly regarded the latter function as the more important, while not at all denying the former. See also p. 64v, and Pagel, *Harvey's Biological Ideas*. pp. 210, 218-19.

184. *PAU*. pp. 74r, 83v, 85r-87r.

185. Ibid., pp. 74r, 81r-83v, 85r-87r.

186. Ibid., p. 87r.

187. Ibid., e.g., pp. 23v, 40v, 43r, 45v, 48v, 49v, 90r, 92r.

188. On the idea that arterial blood is the body's chief nutriment, see Pagel, *Harvey's Biological Ideas*. p. 180 and note 33; p. 199, and note 117; and Bylebyl, "Nutrition, quantification," pp. 371-73, 381-82.

189. *PAU*. p. 11v. See also p. 44v.

190. See ibid., pp. 4r and 5v, where he indicates his intention of dealing with such matters.

191. Ibid., p. 25r; see also p. 40r. On the anti-humoral trend of Harvey's later thought, see Pagel, *New Light on Harvey*. pp. 46-48.

192. Besides the examples given below, see *PAU*., pp. 24v, 25r, 29r, 33v, 34r, 38r, 39r.

193. Ibid., p. 44r.
194. Ibid., pp. 28v, 12r.
195. Ibid., p. 29r.
196. Ibid., p. 39v.
197. Ibid., pp. 39r, 89v, 93r. See also pp. 24v, 35r, 46v, 82r.
198. Ibid., p. 75r. Centralized aggregations of blood were described from the earliest days of the post mortem. See Moritz Roth, *Andreas Vesalius Bruxellensis* (Berlin: Reimer, 1892), p. 5, note 4, quoting a report of 1302: "...dictum Azzolinum ex veneno aliquo mortuum non fuisse, sed potius et certius ex multitudine sanguinis aggregati circa venam magnam...."
199. *PAU.* p. 25r. See also p. 63r.
200. Ibid., pp. 23v-24r, 43v-44v.
201. Ibid., p. 44.
202. Ibid.; see also pp. 41v, 63v.
203. But see ibid., p. 73r, where he refers to an inherent palpitation of the blood in the auricles, and *DMC* ch. 15, p. 60, where he explicitly ascribes to the blood a spontaneous centralizing tendency.
204. *PAU.* p. 44.
205. Ibid., p. 71r. See also p. 86r.
206. Ibid., pp. 77r-80r. On the background to this study, see Pagel, *Harvey's Biological Ideas,* pp. 214-18; Bylebyl, "The growth of *DMC.*" pp. 434-39.
207. *PAU.* p. 79v.
208. Ibid.
209. Ibid., reading "Animi" with the transcript of 1886, rather than "aliis" with Whitteridge. Cf. p. 14r, "Animi pathemata"; *DMC.* p. 45, "animi pathemata"; and Andreas Laurentius, *Historia anatomica* (Paris, 1600), p. 33, "in animi pathematis refugit sanguis ad cor."
210. *PAU.* p. 78v.
211. Ibid., p. 79r.
212. Ibid., p. 78v.
213. *DMC.* ch. 11, p. 48: "Simul etiam de ligaturis manifestum erit, & quare ligaturae attrahunt"; p. 49: "qualis, attractione...usui est"; p. 50: "multam copiam sanguinis affatim attractam esse"; p. 51: "causas attractionis, quae fit per ligaturas"; "attractionem fieri"; "attractionis infra ligaturam." Thus Harvey clearly used the term "attraction" in a purely descriptive sense to refer to the phenomenon of swelling under moderate ligation. At the same time, he made it quite clear (a) that true attraction by heat, pain, and vacuum is inadequate to account for this effect and (b) that the true cause is propulsion by the heart through the arteries. (See especially p. 50, "arteriae...vi & impulsu cordis ab internis corporis partibus foras ultra ligaturam sanguinem trudunt.")
214. See above, p. 57-58.
215. *PAU.* pp. 74r, 79r, 80r.
216. Ibid., p. 80r.
217. This seems especially clear because Fabricius had also made an explicit correlation between the thicker tunics of the arteries and their lack of valves. See above, note 162.
218. *PAU,* pp. 77v and 79r.
219. Harvey's view that the veins would pulsate but for the venous valves shows that he could conceive of the pulse chiefly as an impulse passing through the blood, since the right atrioventricular valve would prevent the heart from propelling any blood into the veins. He must therefore have viewed the arterial pulse as consisting partly in an inflation, but partly in such a transmitted impulse, which could express itself in a copious evacuation when given free reign. For the view of Caspar Hofmann in this regard, see Bylebyl, "Nutrition, quantification," p. 382. See also *DMC* ch. 3, p. 25.
220. Bylebyl, "The growth of *DMC,*" pp. 427-70. See also the critique of Gweneth Whitte-

ridge, *"De motu cordis:* written in two stages?" and my response, *Bull. Hist. Med.,* 1977, *51:* 130-50.

221. Harvey, *DMC,* ch. 8, pp. 41-42. Whitteridge has recently sought to cast doubt on the meaning of Harvey's statement by pointing out that it embodies certain grammatical ambiguities as well as some printer's errors. However, one cannot simply equate grammatical irregularities with semantic obscurity. Even if it does not exactly parse, Harvey's statement conveys the unmistakable message that he first thought of return venous flow as a result of pondering the great quantity of blood transmitted by the heart. See William Harvey, *An Anatomical Disputation Concerning the Movement of the Heart and Blood in Living Creatures,* tr., with intro. and notes by Gweneth Whitteridge (Oxford: Blackwell, 1976), pp. xli-li, and also notes 230 and 242 below.

222. The report by Robert Boyle that Harvey first thought of the circulation through thinking about the valves in the veins, apart from the fact that it is a second-hand account dating from long after the event, seems notably inadequate in this regard, as T. H. Huxley pointed out just a century ago ("William Harvey," pp. 185-88).

223. See above, note 178. Among the phrases Harvey used in this regard was "copia sanguinis," (*PAU,* p. 73r), which was also the key term in his later discussion of the abundance of blood transmitted by the heart (*DMC,* ch. 8, p. 41).

224. Harvey, *PAU,* pp. 77v, 78v, 79r.

225. Ibid., p. 79r.

226. Ibid., p. 79v. The verb "scup" probably alludes to the scupper of a ship, which would be controlled by a leather flap. Harvey later made the point more explicit by reference to "two clacks of a water bellows" (*PAU,* p. 80v).

227. Harvey, Royal Society Notes, #2; repr. in Keynes, *Harvey,* p. 445.

228. The key phrase "copia sanguinis" was commonly used in the medical literature in reference to a pathological excess of blood. For examples, see above, notes 160, 172, and 173. Harvey used the term "copia" in the sense of excess both in his lectures (e.g., p. 29r, "obstructa muccae copia") and in *DMC* (ch. 10, p. 48, "extinctio ob defectum & suffocatio ob copiam").

229. See especially the strongly teleological tone of chapter 17 of *DMC,* which seems to have been written before the discovery of the circulation. See Bylebyl, "The growth of *DMC,"* pp. 446-47, and *"DMC,* two stages," pp. 144-45.

230. "Sane cum copia quanta fuerat." Whitteridge (intro. to her tr. of Harvey, *Movement of the Heart,* pp. xlvii-xlix) chooses not to read this important phrase in the light of the two preceding references to "copia *sanguinis, "* the following, "quanta *scilicet* esset copia transmissi *sanguinis, "* and the repeated references to "copia" or "quantitas *sanguinis* " in the following chapters. She therefore regards "Sane cum copia quanta fuerat" as an ambiguous phrase, and proposes to resolve the ambiguity by inserting the word "inquisitionum" into the text, thus making the discovery stem from "an abundance of *investigations. "* However, even if one were to accept so dubious an approach to textual editing, the unique emphasis on the quantity of the blood would still shine through with unmistakable clarity in the title and whole first paragraph of chapter eight. See Walter Pagel, *New Light on William Harvey,* pp. 3, 5, and also above, notes 223 and 228.

231. *DMC,* ch. 8, p. 41.

232. Bylebyl, "Nutrition, quantification," pp. 378-85.

233. *Nobilium exercitationum libri duodecim de subtilitate* was published at Venice in 1621, but it appears that most of the printing was reissued with a new title page in 1623, together with an appendix, *Par et sanius judicium,* in which Parigiano replied to the criticisms of Mundinus Mundinius. Cf. H. B. Adelmann, *Marcello Malpighi and the Evolution of Embryology,* 5 vols. (Ithaca, N.Y.: Cornell University Press, 1966), V, 2311. I have examined both editions.

234. *De subtilitate,* pp. 267-303.

235. Ibid., p. 297.

236. Bylebyl, "Nutrition, quantification," pp. 378-81.
237. In *De generatione* Ex. 14-16 (*Opera,* pp. 239-48) Harvey discusses pp. 299-303 of Parigiano's book with evident first-hand familiarity. This section follows closely upon Parigiano's quantitative argument (p. 297), and presents an embryological complement to the physiological theory of flux and reflux of arterial blood.
238. Bylebyl, "Nutrition, quantification," pp. 383-84.
239. Bylebyl, *"DMC* two stages," pp. 144-45; and "Nutrition, quantification," pp. 372-74.
240. Compare Harvey's statement with the assertion of Fabricius (above note 160) that but for the valves in the veins, "the blood would have flowed and been attracted to the limbs in such great excess that...either the principal [internal] organs would have been robbed of their nutriment from the vena cava, or the limb vessels would have been in danger of rupture."
241. Harvey repeated this point on p. 44 where he stated that the amount of blood protruded at each beat of the heart is "non parum, cum & ductus non parvi." It was a standard procedure in Galenic teleological anatomy to take the relative size of a vessel as an index of the amount of material that was intended to pass through it. See Galen, *On the Usefulness of the Parts,* e.g., v. 5 and vi. 17; tr. May, I, 256-58, 323-25.
242. Whitteridge has declared that "I do not see how the precise structure of the valves of the heart can have anything whatsoever to do with the abundance of the blood" (intro. to her tr. of *Movement of the Heart,* p. xlviii). However, the connection is made quite clear on p. 43 of *DMC,* where Harvey states as a necessary premise of his hypothetical calculations that the heart protrudes blood in contraction, and added "protrudere enim aliquid semper & ante demonstratum est cap. 3. & omnes in Systole fatentur, ex fabrica valvularum persuasi." A few lines following, he stated, again as a premise in the calculations, that the heart expels some portion of blood at every beat "quae propter impedimentum valvularum in cor remeare non potest." In his letter to Caspar Hofmann of 1636, Harvey again asserted that the quantitative argument depends upon the assumption that the heart transmits some portion of blood at every beat, which can be learned, "ex textura cordis, et valvularum artificio." (Ferrario, Poynter, and Franklin, "William Harvey's debate," p. 15).
243. See the preceding note.
244. *DMC,* ch. 10, p. 47.
245. Above, notes 218 and 219.
246. See above, notes 112 and 118.
247. *DMC,* p. 45, my italics. Furthermore, in both the Proem and chapter 5 of *DMC* (pp. 12-14, 31-32) Harvey made very pointed references to Galen's experimental arteriotomies. If I am correct in maintaining that these portions of the treatise predate the discovery of the circulation, then this would show that a certain preoccupation with Galen's observations was an actual precondition of the discovery. See above, note 220.
248. *DMC,* p. 45: "Arterias autem nullibi sanguinem e venis recipere, nisi transmissione facta per cor." Cf. also p. 46: "de venis in arteriis nullibi datur transitus, nisi per cor ipsum, & per pulmones"; and p. 53: "arteriae nusquam sanguinem e venis recipiunt nisi e sinistro ventriculo cordis." The reiteration bespeaks a certain preoccupation with opposing Galen in this point, and again the early sections of *DMC* give reason to suppose that this attitude predated the discovery of the circulation. See Bylebyl, "The growth of *DMC,"* pp. 458-60.
249. One could reasonably surmise such familiarity simply from the fact that Harvey was a well-educated physician, but again the early chapters of *DMC* provide explicit confirmation of such prior knowledge. For in defending the pulmonary transit in chapter 7, p. 38, Harvey quoted the following statement from Galen: "In toto est mutua Anastomosis, atque oscillorum apertio arteriis simul cum venis, transumuntque ex sese pariter sanguinem, & spiritum per invisibiles quasdam atque augustas plane vias." See also *DMC,* ch. 12, p. 53, "videmus enim ab arteriis sanguinem in venas dimanare, non e venis in arterias," and compare with the preceding note. See also Harvey's letter to P. M. Slegel of 1651 (*Opera,* p. 616): "Medici omnes rationales olim

nuperque crediderunt dari mutuam quandam sanguinis transvasationem, sive accessum et recessum inter venas et arterias; ejusque rei causa, anastomoses passim invisibiles (nempe apertiones quasdam inconspicuas, sive occulta foramina) effinxerunt, per quae sanguis huc illuc flueret, atque e vase in vas migraret et remigraret."

250. As is well known, in *DMC* Harvey took no definite stand as to the actual nature of the connections between arteries and veins. At one point (p. 46) he stated, "with regard to the anastomosis of veins and arteries, where, how, and for what reason it occurs, one might suspect that no one has had anything correct to say. I am currently engaged in studying this matter." Elsewhere (p. 48) he stated that "in the parts and extremities the blood passes from the arteries into the veins either directly through the anastomoses, or indirectly through the porosities of the flesh, or in both ways." However, even from such brief statements we learn two important points: First, any consideration of the passage of blood from arteries into veins is founded upon the traditional doctrine of anastomoses, whether or not the ultimate result of the inquiry is to confirm the specific details of the latter doctrine. Second, Harvey did not see it as crucially important to his case for the circulation to resolve this particular issue—he could casually put it off to the indefinite future, apparently comfortable in the belief that no one would challenge him on these particular grounds. For Harvey's later views on the anastomoses, see Yehuda Elkuna and June Goodfield, "Harvey and the problem of the 'capillaries,' " *Isis,* 1968, *59:* 61-73.

251. On all these points, see above, pp. 46-51, 58-59, 63.

252. *DMC,* chs. 11 & 12, esp. pp. 52-54.

253. I.e., a normal rush of blood from the arteries into the veins, and a normal rush of blood from the veins into the heart, and so on to the arteries.

254. *DMC,* pp. 55-56.

255. Ibid., ch. 11, pp. 48-53. See also above notes 89 and 96.

256. Ibid., pp. 51-52.

257. Ibid., p. 48; see also pp. 55-56, 60.

258. Ibid., p. 42. For background, see Pagel, *Harvey's Biological Ideas,* pp. 89-119, esp. 90-93 and 104 n. 66: and *New Light on William Harvey,* pp. 76-77.

259. *DMC,* p. 41.

260. Pagel, *Harvey's Biological Ideas,* passim, esp. pp. 82-124; *New Light,* pp. 20-21, 37-41.

261. Webster, "William Harvey and the crisis of medicine in Jacobean England," pp. 15-23. above.

262. These continuities have been pointed out by L. J. Rather, "Old and new views of the emotions and bodily changes: Wright and Harvey versus Descartes, James and Cannon," *Clio Medica,* 1966, *1:* 5-8.

263. *DMC,* p. 60.

264. Ibid., my italics.

265. Fabricius, *De venarum ostiolis,* ed. Franklin, p. 73.

266. Ibid., pp. 52, 74.

267. *DMC,* p. 61. The cause of the periodicity of fevers was a subject much discussed by Harvey's immediate predecessors and contemporaries. See Santorio, *Commentaria in primam sectionem Aphorismorum Hippocratis* (Venice, 1629), cols. 245-51. On the related issue of the inward movement of drugs and poisons, see Pagel, *New Light,* pp. 147-51.

268. See above, pp. 67, 69.

269. For Harvey's later use of the term in the sense of "period," see Pagel, *Harvey's Biological Ideas,* pp. 84-85.

270. For example, the index of Jean Fernel, *Opera medicinalia* (Venice, 1566) has one entry under *circuitus,* namely "circuituum quae causa sit. 307." This refers to *Pathologia,* iv. 11, whose title is, "Quae circuituum causa sit, & quid eorum ordinem formamque mutet." It is clearly assumed that the reader will recognize the technical meaning of the term in relation to intermittent fevers.

271. *DMC.* pp. 44–45.

272. E.g., F. R. Jevons, "Harvey's quantitative method," *Bull. Hist. Med..* 1962, *36:* 462–67. Pagel, *Harvey's Biological Ideas.* p. 73, also takes issue with Jevons on this point.

273. In fact, in *DMC.* ch. 12, p. 54, Harvey describes how, in consequence of strong emotion and other factors, the heart's transmission of blood might be reduced to a minimal, "drop by drop *(guttatim)"* basis. Whether by coincidence or not, his opponents invoked the idea of a *normal* "drop by drop" transmission to elude the force of the quantitative argument. See Bylebyl, "Nutrition, quantification," pp. 383–84 and note 58; and Pagel, *Harvey's Biological Ideas.* pp. 74–76.

The Image of Harvey
in Commonwealth and Restoration England

Robert G. Frank, Jr.

After William Harvey's death in 1657, his friend, the M.D. and poet Abraham Cowley, composed an "Ode Upon Dr. Harvey" that epitomized in five stanzas the physiologist's accomplishments in the eyes of his younger colleagues.[1] Harvey was Apollo, passionately pursuing truth, the nymph Daphne: "Coy Nature, (which remain'd, though Aged grown,/A Beauteous virgin still, injoyd by none,/Nor even unveil'd by any one)." With sharp eyes Harvey traced his Daphne through "winding streams of blood," into the very heart itself,

> And held this slippery *Proteus* in a chain,
> Till all her mighty Mysteries she descry'd
> Which from his wit the attempt before to hide
> Was the first Thing that Nature did in vain.

Nor could the "young Practise of New life," whether it "in the womb or egg be wrought," conceal its secrets from Harvey's surveying eyes.

> Thus Harvey sought for truth in truths own Book
> The creatures, which by God himself was writ;
> And wisely thought 'twas fit,
> Not to read Comments only upon it,
> But on th' original it self to look.

Harvey had cured the very art of curing, purged it of old errors, freed it of all inveterate diseases. He would have disclosed yet more secrets, had not his loyalty to the king, and "a Barba'rous Wars unlearned Rage" destroyed his remaining works.

Thus Cowley saw the elements of Harvey's life: unrelenting dissection, exploration of the heart, the discovery of the circulation, the delineation of embryonic growth, all leading to the overthrow of the ancients—accomplishments ill-rewarded by Harvey's suffering and the loss of his manuscripts.

Cowley's poem, like all rhetorical pieces, deliberately combined fact, metaphor, and value judgment to create an image in some senses larger than life—a myth or symbol. Every great life and achievement is the potential subject matter of myth, and amenable to transformation into symbol; Harvey's proved more so than most. In this paper I wish to examine the emergence, nature, and function of Harvey as myth and symbol, from the 1650s through the 1680s, that is, in the last years of Harvey's life and those immediately following his death. Since the mythopoeic or symbolic content of a man's life consists, by definition, in a systematized perception that transcends the narrow boundaries of his actual accomplishments, I shall perforce look beyond the confines of books on anatomy, physiology, and learned medicine. To be sure, a Harveian tradition existed there as well, but it cannot be explored within the short compass of a single paper. Rather, I wish to look at the *pattern of popular acceptance* and the *substance of popular perception*—the "reputation" or "image"—of Harvey and his discoveries in England during the Commonwealth and Restoration periods.

I shall first sketch out, very briefly and more as background than as an object of analysis, the great growth of anatomical endeavors in England from approximately 1640 to 1660, emphasizing the centrality of Harvey to this change. From the crucial period of the 1650s I shall present evidence of the acceptance of Harvey's work at Oxford and Cambridge. I shall explore the pattern and content of growing esteem for Harvey at the College of Physicians in the 1650s and 1660s, and how this focused on the institutions of the Harveian Museum and Harveian Orations. I shall show how, during this same period, Harvey's name and accomplishments were presented to the public in a variety of ways, through literary works written by both physicians and non-physicians. Thus, it is not surprising that, during the period ca. 1665-1685, physicians used this public image of Harvey specifically, and that of the anatomical physician generally, in polemical works designed to defend their intellectual preeminence and professional privileges. Lest one think that praise for the Harveian image was unanimous, I shall also examine some attacks made during the same period both on Harvey and on the tradition of the anatomical physician. Finally, I shall close with some generalizations about the nature and function of mythologies in science, and most especially in the early modern medical sciences.

Background: The Growth of English Anatomy, 1640–1660

When Harvey published *De motu cordis* in 1628, he was very much an oddity in English medical life: a physician who advanced the science of medicine as well as practiced its art. This was not because England lacked either numerous physicians or medical authors. Since the mid-sixteenth century, the numbers of university-trained physicians had more than quadrupled, with the largest growth in London, and to a lesser degree in the university towns of Oxford and Cambridge. A growing proportion of these physicians had been educated in the famous medical schools of the Continent, especially at Padua and Leyden. In London, Harvey's beloved College of Physicians organized the medical elite of the metropolis, and even provided a modicum of continuing education in the form of occasional anatomies and Harvey's own Lumleian lectures. A significant number of collegiate and university physicians were authors of a wide range of scholarly and popular books in medicine, the sciences, and belles lettres.[2] English medicine by 1628 lacked only the crucial ingredient: a tradition of original investigation, carried forward by a body of medical scientists, especially anatomists, who extended scientific knowledge rather than merely using it.

That changed rapidly in the succeeding three decades.[3] By 1660 English medicine could number among its glories no less than seven anatomists known throughout Europe. Harvey's *De motu cordis* (1628), *De circulatione* (1649) and *De generatione* (1651) led the way. George Ent skillfully defended Harvey and the circulation in his *Apologia pro circulatione sanguinis* (1641). Francis Glisson's *De rachitide* (1650) and *Anatomia hepatis* (1654) showed both the clinical and scientific sides of his talent. Nathaniel Highmore's *Corporis humani disquisitio anatomica* (1651) was the first English anatomical textbook to support Harvey, while in his *History of Generation* (1651) he supplemented Harvey's findings on the same subject. Thomas Wharton's *Adenographia* (1656) did for the glands what his mentor, Glisson, had done for the liver. Walter Charleton's *Oeconomia animalis* (1659) became a standard European textbook in physiology, while Thomas Willis's *Diatribae duae* (1659), on fermentation and fever, applied chemistry and anatomy to clinical problems.

Beyond these anatomists and physiologists whose work was published before the Restoration, one may discern another group of more than a dozen men researching anatomical problems, but whose findings came into print later, or in some cases of mischance, not at all. Charles Scarburgh, Jonathan Goddard, Christopher Merrett, Daniel Whistler, George Joyliffe, William Petty, and Henry Power all began their investigatory careers in the 1640s. They were followed in the 1650s by Robert Boyle, Ralph Bathurst, Henry Clerke, Philip Stephens, Timothy Clarke, Walter Needham, Christopher Wren, Christopher Terne, and Richard Tower. The chronological pattern of

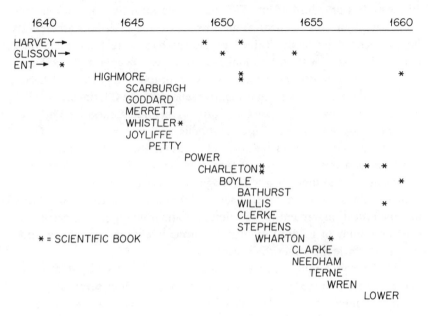

Fig. 1. The entry of English physicians into anatomical research.

entry of these physicians into original research, and their resultant publications, is shown in Figure 1.

These almost two dozen anatomists worked in many milieus—some in the Schools and college rooms of Oxford and Cambridge, others in London lodgings and at the College of Physicians. Clusters of them knew each others' work intimately, and they were associated with each other as colleagues at university or at the College of Physicians, as teacher and student, or as collaborators in joint research, discussion, and correspondence. The network of their relationships more resembles the web of a spider than the neat branching trees of intellectual genealogy sometimes drawn for nineteenth-century scientists.

In ways too intricate to specify here, this network had its origin in Harvey. In London in the late 1630s and early 1640s, at Oxford during the siege in 1642–46, and even in the relative isolation imposed upon him by political circumstances during the Commonwealth, Harvey built up a coterie of followers. Disciples like Glisson, Ent, Highmore, Scarburgh, Charleton, and Merrett, in turn had associates and students of their own. All felt, in varying degrees, and for varying lengths of time in their careers, inspired by Harvey's accomplishment, attracted by the scientific problems it left unsolved, and inclined to direct their own work according to the canons of unflagging dissection and careful experimentation explicit in Harvey's writing and teaching. A schematic representation of these relationships is given in Figure 2.

Perhaps just as important for the later development of English science, these anatomists did not emulate the solitary fashion in which Harvey had conducted the research that led to *De motu cordis*. They banded together for experimentation and discussion. Harvey himself worked with a number of them—we know for certain Highmore and Scarburgh—during his Oxford sojourn. One of the precursors of the Royal Society, the London "1645 Group" mentioned in the recollections of the mathematician John Wallis, included a core of anatomical physicians. Individual and cooperative research projects in anatomy and clinical medicine abounded at the College of Physicians during the late 1640s and throughout the 1650s. The Oxford philosophical club in the 1650s, although its agenda was built primarily around topics in the physical sciences, included a stalwart group of physicians who were anatomists and chemists. When the Royal Society was founded in 1660, it recruited its member physicians from all of these precursors.

The effects of these changes in the personnel, organization, and productivity of the English medical community may be seen most vividly in charting the publications of British anatomy (Figure 3). Works published in the late sixteenth and early seventeenth centuries were few in number, and largely reprints of continental editions. By the late seventeenth century, books in anatomy by British authors had not only grown phenomenally in numbers, but were often reprinted on the continent, thus reversing (or at least equilibrating) the intellectual balance of trade.

The Acceptance of Harvey at Oxford and Cambridge

But to extend the influence of Harvey's discoveries beyond a handful of cognoscenti anatomists, it was necessary for his fame to spread into the "hatcheries" of the English intelligentsia, the two ancient universities. Aubrey said of Harvey's circulation that "with much adoe at last, in about 20 or 30 yeares time, it was received in all the Universities in the world."[4] What was true of the world was true of Oxford and Cambridge.

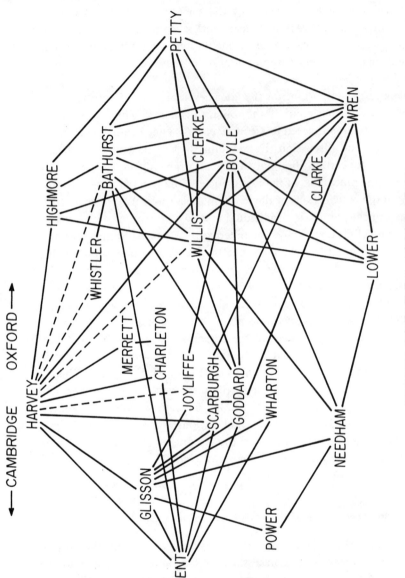

← CAMBRIDGE   OXFORD →

——— = KNOWN SCIENTIFIC ASSOCIATION

‑ ‑ ‑ = PROBABLE SCIENTIFIC RELATIONSHIP

Fig. 2. The network of Harvey's English disciples.

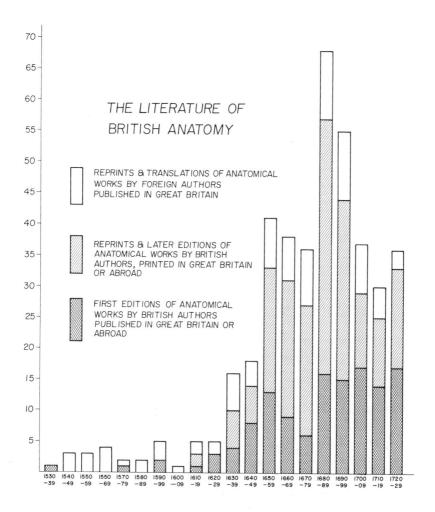

Fig. 3. Publications in British anatomy, 1530–1720.

Glisson, as Regius Professor of Medicine at Cambridge from 1636 to 1677, was most instrumental in introducing Harvey into their home university. On the basis of some misinterpreted evidence, and from his absenteeism after the Restoration, it is often assumed that Glisson resided away from Cambridge almost from the beginning, and treated his Professorship as a sinecure.[5] Nothing could be farther from the truth; before the 1660s he seems to have divided his time between terms in Cambridge and vacations in London. Moreover, among the fifteen fat volumes of his manuscripts in the British Library are over 400 separate orations, lectures, and disputations on anatomy, physiology, and medicine, the great bulk of which seem to be ascribable to his teaching duties.[6] Most of the lectures were on clinical subjects, but scattered among these are a large number on anatomy and physiology, including items on the heart, lungs, arteries, and veins.[7] Many lectures were straight from the Harveian corpus: "On the Circuit of the Blood"; "The Arteries Are Moved According to the Motion of the Heart"; "The Primitive Motion of the Blood is Intrinsic"; "The Ideas of Descartes Concerning the Motion of the Heart are not Consonant with the Truth"; as well as a number of untitled lecture notes on the motion of the blood that included answers to objections.[8] The origin and properties of the blood interested Glisson no less than its movement. He lectured on how "There are No Vital Spirits Separable from the Blood," how "In Every Fever There Is a Fermentation of the Blood," that "The Blood is the Cause of Sanguification," and that "Blood Alone is the Innate Heat."[9] Examples could be multiplied manyfold. There were lectures on embryology, animal heat, the functions of the spleen, liver, stomach, lacteals, and lymphatics.

The same innovative spirit may be seen in the topics disputed by students at Cambridge with Glisson as *praeses*. As a student, Wallis was interested in "the speculative part of *Physick* and *Anatomy*," and about 1640 was the first of Glisson's "Sons, who (in a publick Disputation) maintain'd the Circulation of the Bloud, (which was then a new Doctrine)."[10] Medical students did similar disputations, and although the great majority of those done under Glisson were understandably on such clinical topics as fevers, phlebotomy, purgation, diet, and medication, by the 1650s a significant portion of the respondents answered on topics in the new anatomy and physiology. One young doctor recapitulated how "The Blood is Moved in a Circle."[11] In 1653 the man who later became Glisson's deputy and successor, Robert Brady, enumerated the evidence why "The Pulsation of the Arteries is Caused by the Impulsion of Blood from the Heart."[12] Glisson's own interest in the liver found reflection in student theses. In 1652 Joyliffe argued the proposition that "The Separation of Bile is the Proper Function of the Liver."[13] In 1654 Henry Power debated the complementary thesis, that "The Liver is Not the Organ of Sanguification," as the Galenic tradition had held.[14] Similar examples may be adduced from the late 1650s: on the spleen as a source of a sanguinary ferment, on the blood as a principal part, on its role in nutrition, and on the function of respiration. All were based firmly on the circulation and its implications.

Among Glisson's students at Cambridge, Henry Power is a particularly interesting example of Harveian influences exerted at a distance.[15] In the late 1640s he followed his friend Thomas Browne's advice to learn anatomy by *autopsia*, and most especially to make himself master of Harvey's *De motu cordis*.[16] By 1652 his reading, and dissections on a large number of animals, led Power to compose a small tract, "Circulatio sanguinis."[17] The manuscript brought forward over fifty experiments, both dissectional and vivisectional (including one later published by Glisson), to support "our Reverend and Worthy Dr. Harvey," and "that incomparable Invention of his, the Circulation of the Blood"[18]—a sentiment that seems to have been shared by Power's fellow students at Cambridge in the 1650s.

Oxford, though it lacked a Glisson to put forward Harvey's cause, had had the physiologist himself, if only briefly, in 1642-1646. After the siege was lifted, there was something of a hiatus when most of Harvey's known colleagues in the university town were dispersed: George Bathurst died in 1644, and the Regius, Thomas Clayton, Sr., in 1647; Scarburgh, Highmore, John Greaves, Cowley, Merrett, Charleton and Joyliffe had all left Oxford by 1648. Only the younger medicos, Willis, Ralph Bathurst and Edward Greaves, stayed on. But these proved to be quite sufficient, especially when reinforced in the early 1650s, with the arrival from London of men like Petty, Goddard and Boyle, and with the recruitment of such locals as Henry Clerke, Timothy Clarke and Christopher Wren.

Rapid change began with the brief sojourn of that scientist-entrepreneur, William Petty. When he arrived in Oxford in 1649, he was already well disposed to Harveianism; he had studied with Jan van der Wale and Cornelius van Hooghelande in the Netherlands, and had carried out anatomical research of his own at Paris and London in the late 1640s.[19] Before departing in late 1652 for more remunerative adventures in Ireland, Petty had organized a club of local experimental philosophers (including Wallis, Bathurst, Clerke, and Willis) to meet at his lodgings;[20] one of their exploits, the resuscitation of a hanged woman destined for the anatomical table, gained for Petty the university's Tomlins Readership in Anatomy.[21] He used these Oxford lectures to preach the mix of Harveian physiology and Cartesian philosophy he had learned in the Netherlands.[22] For example, Petty began his public lecture at the Act in 1651 by reciting a poem in praise of Harvey and his work.[23] His anatomical lectures similarly slighted the statutory injunction to teach descriptive anatomy in the Galenic mold, and concentrated instead on theories concerning the motion of the heart, the function of respiration, and the origin of the blood.[24]

As at Cambridge, medical disputations in the 1650s and 1660s too reflected changing physiological allegiances. In the 1630s these university exercises had dealt largely with clinical matters such as therapy and diet; one respondent affirmed that beer was more beneficial in fevers than barley water, while another argued that every pleurisy had four phases.[25] When disputing began in 1651, its face had changed. At the Act that year, while Petty praised Harvey in verse, Bathurst argued that the foetus was not nourished by the maternal blood, and drew his arguments directly from *De generatione*, published just a few months before.[26] In 1652 another medical student denied that chyle was brought to the liver, a thesis most certainly based on Pecquet's discovery of the thoracic duct the year before.[27] In 1653 Timothy Clarke rejected the notion that sanguification took place in the liver, spleen, or veins, and a colleague defended three theses straight out of *De generatione:* that there were no spirits distinct from the blood, that all animals originated from an egg, and that the foetus sucked in the uterus.[28] In the following decade disputations continued to take the same Harveian lines of speculation: that rickets might be caused by obstructed circulation, that respiration depurated the blood, that the circulation of the blood took place through the lungs, that the four humors did not make up the blood, and that the liver was not its manufactory.[29]

Even at the beginning of their careers, Oxford medical students learned anatomy with a Harveian bent. During the 1650s the head of Hart Hall, Philip Stephens, taught tutorial groups from Johannes Vesling's *Syntagma anatomicum*, a popular introductory text.[30] More importantly, Vesling was a correspondent of Harvey, and his book was one of the few student manuals that accepted the circulation.[31] Vesling described the motions of the heart, the structure of its valves, and explained that since the heart continuously sent out blood to the periphery to replenish the vital heat and spirits of the parts, it must necessarily return to the heart in a perpetual circular motion.[32] It was to the assiduity of William Harvey, Vesling said, that we owed, for the first time in this age, the more exact knowledge of these things.[33]

Everywhere in the university town one may find evidence of Harvey's acceptance. In 1654 Seth Ward agreed with critic John Webster's praise of Harvey's circulation, and of recent progress in anatomy, but pointed out that one could not expect such advances in the theory of medicine to change the day-to-day practice of medicine radically. In any case, Ward said, it was the learned physicians, rather than Webster's empirics, who had mastered medical practice; had not Dr. Harvey performed "cures of desperate Ulcers and diseases, even of the Cancer."[34] The biggest Oxford bookseller, Richard Davis, carried all of Harvey's works, both in Latin and English, as well as those of his English followers Ent, Glisson, Highmore, Charleton, and Willis.[35] Many of the libraries of dons, especially those connected to the Oxford "Clubb" of experimental philosophers, had Harvey's works. These included divines such as Richard Allestree[36] and John Owen,[37] as well as physicians like Ralph Bathurst,[38] John Locke,[39] Henry Stubbe,[40] and William Levinz.[41] Even a gentleman commoner such as Robert Southwell, when he left Oxford for the grand tour in 1659-1661, was cognizant enough of Harvey's discoveries to note, when in Rome, an unresolved query that had been put to Harvey by an Italian anatomist.[42]

In sum, many separate lines of evidence suggest that by the late 1640s and early 1650s, Harvey's discoveries were well known to both teachers and students at the English universities, and were rapidly becoming the mold for a recasting of the basic medical sciences of anatomy and physiology, a task of a magnitude unsurpassed since Galen.

The Image of Harvey at the Royal College of Physicians

Both the accelerating pace of anatomical research and the exposure of university students to Harvey's name and accomplishments were consolidated into a larger public perception of Harvey by the Royal College of Physicians of London. This process is particularly interesting because it was not without its ups and downs.

In the 1610s, 1620s, and 1630s, as Keynes and Webster have demonstrated, Harvey was an active, respected, and highly influential member of the college. He frequently attended meetings at Amen Corner, and vigorously carried out his duties as an Elect, as Lumleian Lecturer, sometimes as censor, and often as a member of special committees.[43] But his high status had nothing to do with his anatomical discoveries. Almost the opposite was true. Aubrey reported that because of *De motu cordis,* the vulgar thought him "crack-brained" and Harvey "fell mightily in his Practize," while "all the physitians were against his Opinion."[44] Although Harvey claimed that he had frequently demonstrated to his fellow Collegians the truth of his findings,[45] only Robert Fludd among them praised the circulation at this time.[46] James Primrose attacked Harvey's work vehemently,[47] and the remainder of the College maintained a prudent silence. College lectures by Glisson and Ent in 1639-1642 seem to have accepted the circulation,[48] but the College as a whole preferred not to be drawn into the controversy; as late as 1641 it refused either to approve or to condemn the tract of a recent Leyden graduate, Roger Drake, defending Harvey's circulation against Primrose's attack.[49]

For the next ten years Harvey did not attend a meeting at the College,[50] and became increasingly estranged from its activities. His position as Physician-in-Ordinary to Charles I bound him to the king's cause, and Harvey's fortunes declined with those of the monarch. Ent, visiting Harvey in December 1647, found him dismayed with political events.[51] His request in 1648 to attend the imprisoned king was refused. In 1650 Harvey required Parliamentary permission even to enter London to attend a patient. On the Continent he was rumoured to be dead, and an admiring Dutchman even composed a premature threnody.[52]

The College had also changed in the interim; as Sharp has recently pointed out, it came to be greatly influenced, even if not dominated, by physicians who were closely linked to the Parliamentary cause.[53] John Clarke, its president in the late 1640s, had in 1643 used government influence to do the absent Harvey out of his place as Physician to St. Bartholomew's Hospital.[54] One almost feels that the College was generous in granting Harvey sufference to sue for his Lumleian arrears,[55] and did not instead, as it had in the case of other Royalist physicians, use non-attendance as an excuse for depriving him entirely.

Harvey's repute began to rise again in the 1650s. This change was no doubt partly political. Harvey's old friend Francis Prujean was elected President in 1650. Harvey's movements were no longer restricted; insofar as his advanced age allowed, he visited London, attended some College meetings, and made friends with a number of younger virtuosi, such as John Aubrey and Robert Boyle, and an older one, Thomas Hobbes.[56] Each passing year since the king's execution made his former retainers seem less dangerous.

The magnitude of Harvey's scientific accomplishment also came increasingly to the fore. Goddard, in his College lectures in 1647, had praised recent discoveries in anatomy.[57] Baldwin Hamey's lectures of 1648 had been explicitly based on the circulation, as had Richard Catcher's of 1649.[58] Ent brought out Harvey's *De generatione* in 1651, which rapidly went through several printings in Latin and English. The incumbents of College lectureships in the early 1650s—Glisson, Wharton, Joyliffe, Merrett—were Harveian partisans, and seem to have based their presentations on his discoveries.[59]

Harvey, a childless widower, personally extended that influence by taking steps to insure that the College itself would be his heir. In 1651 the College unanimously accepted Harvey's anonymous offer, tendered by Prujean, to construct a new wing to house a library and meeting room.[60] The Harveian Museum, described by Aubrey as "a noble building of Roman Architecture" with Corinthian pillasters,[61] was opened in Harvey's presence in 1654, complete with speeches by Prujean and Ent.[62] Soon thereafter, Merrett was made Librarian, and in Harvey's will he bequeathed to the College what books and papers Scarburgh and Ent might think fit, and which had not already been transferred there.[63]

One may get a sense of the size and nature of the Harveian Museum from a catalogue published by Merrett in 1660, before the entire College was destroyed in the Great Fire of 1666.[64] It was an uncompromisingly professional library, with no works in logic, theology, or general literature. The 1280 titles in medicine, the medical sciences, and natural philosophy were overwhelmingly continental in origin, and less than two dozen were in languages other than Latin. As one might expect, over half of the titles were on the clinical side. But the library also contained—perhaps here reflecting Harvey's contributions—a magnificent collection of anatomical works by sixteenth and early seventeenth-century authors. Even a partial list reads almost like a bibliography to Harvey's Lumleian Lectures: Berengario da Carpi, Vesalius, Etienne, Colombo, Massa, Eustachio, Platter, Fallopio, Piccolomini, Valverde, Bauhin, Du Laurens, Fabricius ab Aquapendente, and Hofmann.[65] The library also contained relatively few anatomical and physiological works from the 1640s and 1650s, again reflecting Harvey's declining interest in anatomical literature during the latter part of his life. It had seven works of Harvey's supporter and fellow Collegian, the Rosicrucian Robert Fludd, as well as one of Harvey's opponent, Emilio Parigiano.[66] There was a respectable number of works by modern astronomers and natural philosophers, including Copernicus, Kepler, Galileo, Descartes, Gilbert and Digby, but the presumption is rather less strong that these were Harvey's.[67] There was also a large collection of about eight dozen surgical and dissecting instruments and an about equal number of "Res Curiosae & Exoticae"—mostly preserved animal specimens.[68] The entire collection of books and objects was most likely displayed in glass-fronted presses lining the walls, probably more than a dozen in number. The library was a fitting memorial to Harvey, whose benefaction the College commemorated by erecting a white marble bust, with an inscription praising his discoveries on the motion of the blood and on the origin of animals.[69]

Mutual cordialities did not stop there. In September 1654 the College elected him President, an honor he declined for reasons of age and health.[70] Harvey reciprocated in June and July of 1656 by making over to the College an estate to endow a yearly feast and oration. Annually on this occasion benefactors were to be praised and the fellows exhorted both to mutual love and affection, and "to search and studdy out the secrett of Nature by way of Experiment."[71]

The College was true to Harvey's intentions. Until the destruction of the College by the Great Fire intermitted the Orations for a dozen years, its members gathered annually to dine, to hear benefactors praised, and to be exhorted to follow an investigator's way. The list of Harveian Orators from 1656 to 1665 includes many—such as Edmund Wilson, Daniel Whistler, Thomas Coxe and Nathan Paget—who must have known Harvey well, and one—Charles Scarburgh—who knew him intimately. So it is little surprising that when the Orators came to praise benefactors, they singled out Harvey.

Several of these Orations are extant in print or in manuscript, and give some sense of the way Harvey's exemplar was held continually before the Fellowship. In 1657 Edmund Wilson used the occasion to praise Harvey especially, and to give an account of his death.[72] In 1661 a veteran of the Oxford siege, Sir Edward Greaves, first recounted the dignities of the medical profession, and then spent most of the Oration praising Harvey's anatomical accomplishments, genius, liberality, good fellowship, and service to the College; even though Harvey's splendid library and benefactions were worthy of praise, in his discoveries on the circulation and on generation, Greaves said, Harvey had erected his own best monument.[73] Greaves even took the occasion to dismiss in passing the spurious priority claims of Caesalpinus and Hofmann.[74]

In the following year Scarburgh praised Harvey by speaking more intimately about the physiologist.[75] He told of Harvey's assiduousness in his studies, and of his Continental travels. He commended Harvey's integrity in believing that *De motu cordis* should stand or fall solely on the merits of its experiments. Scarburgh lauded other English experimental philosophers, such as Gilbert, Bacon, and Digby, and commended the contributions made to anatomical studies by Fellows of the College. He told of the breadth of Harvey's investigations, gave a list of his lost treatises, and condemned the havoc that had destroyed them. Scarburgh even hinted that Harvey had hoped to set up a professorship of experimental philosophy at Cambridge, but was deterred by its reputation as a haven for radicals and heretics. Most of all, Scarburgh praised Harvey's personal and scientific character: his simplicity, his humility, and his ability to grasp the essentials of any question.[76] Clearly Scarburgh, as Greaves before him, saw the Oration not merely as a general celebration of benefactors, but as an occasion to clarify, define, and defend the memory of the College's most illustrious member.

Harvey in Commonwealth and Early Restoration Literature

Many who knew of Harvey and his accomplishments, both physician and non-physician alike, were not content merely to see him memorialized in stone at the College, or praised there intramurally. Beginning in the early 1650s, Harvey's name and his achievements are to be found with increasing frequency in works of poetry, history, theology, and philosophy written either by litterateurs, or by physicians with literary avocations.

On the most elementary level, Harvey's findings entered into literary works as facts that could be adduced to support one or another kind of argument, or as the foundation for rhetorical flights of fancy. In a poem written to Brian Duppa, bishop of Salisbury, the Christ Church divine William Cartwright referred obliquely to a "circling of Actions, as of Bloud;/Motion as in a Mill/Is busie standing still."[77] When this and other poems were published posthumously in 1651, Sir John Berkenhead, a fellow of All Souls as well as a journalist and courtier, in turn praised Cartwright's wit by comparing it to Harvey's circulation: *"For as immortall* HARVEY'S *searching Brain/Found the* Red Spirit's *Circle in each Veyn,"* so did Cartwright's wit prove *"its* Circulation *through all Arts."*[78] In a long poem of 1658, Francis Vernon praised Oxford as a place where the physician obtained:

> His knowledge in the *Mystery* of the *veins*
> And *nervs;* of late his *skill* he so inhances
> By finding out the *blood's Maeandring dances,*
> That he *old nature* with Industrious pain
> Renews, makes *aged AEson* young again.[79]

In the following year another young Oxford poet, Thomas Sprat, versified the saga of the Athenian plague, including vivid descriptions of how the disease tainted the blood and invaded the thorax. Therefore "That which before was natures noblest Art,/The circulation from the heart,/Was most destructfull now," because it speeded poisoned blood to every part.[80] Interestingly, all concerned had a direct or indirect connection to Harvey; Duppa, Cartwright, and Berkenhead were at Oxford with Harvey during the siege, while Vernon and Sprat were privy to the activities of the Oxford experimental philosophy club in the 1650s.

Another friend from the Oxford siege, Walter Charleton,[81] used Harvey's findings in theological works. In a tract against atheism of 1652, Charleton sketched the gradations of life, and gave facts about oysters gleaned by "our *Democritus Londinensis*, that incomparable indagator of Nature's Arcana, Dr. *Harvey.*"[82] In discussing *fortuna* Charleton once again had recourse to Harvey's authority, this time on the question of scientific serendipity: "We have it from the pen of that oraculous Secretary of Nature, Dr. *Harvey*, that he never dissected any Animal, but he always discovered somthing or other more then he expected, nay then ever he thought on before; so useful & infinite in variety is the *Magna Charta* of *Nature.*"[83]

Charleton likewise referred to Harvey five years later in another theological tract, this time on the soul's immortality.[84] In a lengthy digression Charleton described investigative science at Oxford, and especially at the College of Physicians,[85] where there were those "who daily investigate arguments to confirm and advance that incomparable invention of Doctor *Harvey*, the *Circulation of the Blood.*"[86] These anatomists had brought the doctrine of the circulation to such a high degree of perfection that many difficult questions of pathology could be resolved using only that hypothesis. Not only diagnosis, but therapy, had been thereby so much improved that Charleton was considering undertaking "to justify all the Aphorisms of Hippocrates, which concern the Nature and Sanation of Diseases, by reasons and considerations deduced meerly from this one Fountain, the Hypothesis of the Circulation of the blood."[87] Not content to praise just the circulation, Charleton later introduced Harvey's work on generation, and used it to support his contention that the blood was "the *Common Medium, Cement* or Glew" that united body and soul. "Our perspicacious Countryman" had proved in his *De generatione* that blood was the part of the body first created, and that therefore it circulated perpetually "like a river of *Living water*," irrigating the substance of all parts and communicating to them both heat and life. The soul, Charleton believed, was "an intimate Praesence" in this blood.[88] Much the same point came up again in another of Charleton's moral works written in 1664. In discussing the nature of wit he affirmed again that the blood was the fountain of natural heat, life and invigoration; thus, "Dr. *Harvey*, somewhere in his Book of the *Generation of Animals*, affirms it to be no small advantage to the Brain, that Students and contemplative Men preserve their mass of Blood pure and uncorrupt."[89]

The philosopher Henry More provides another interesting example of Harvey's facts cropping up in the oddest places. In his case, as in that of Charleton, there are some probable reasons. The Cambridge don was patronized by one of Harvey's patients, Lady Anne Conway, and may even have met Harvey in the 1650's.[90] Certainly More knew enough of Harvey's work by 1659 to appeal to the findings of "that judicious Naturalist Dr.

Harvey" in a passage discussing the effects of the soul on monstrous births.[91] Sometime in the next two decades, most probably in the 1660s, More was sufficiently inspired by reading *De motu cordis* to write a Latin epic poem praising Harvey's discoveries and recapitulating the arguments for the circulation of the blood.[92] He explained in detail how the heart pumped more blood than could be supplied by the ingesta, how ligatures show that blood entered a limb by the arteries and left by the veins, how circulating blood carried heat to all parts, how the valves in the veins pointed towards the heart, how the structure of the heart showed that it pumped blood through the lungs, and how, in the embryo, the circulation bypassed the lungs. Appropriately, More ended with Harvey's conclusion: the heart moved the blood throughout the whole body, never allowing it to stagnate.[93] All of this was expressed in 106 dense and florid lines of Latin dactylic hexameter. One rather wonders if Harvey would have appreciated quite so much attention from the Cambridge philosopher.

Other litterateurs chose to emphasize, not Harvey's factual discoveries, but his role as a long-suffering public benefactor. In his *Worthies of England* (1662), Thomas Fuller gave a capsule biography and assessment of Harvey's contributions. Harvey was "not only *Doctor Medicinae,* but *Doctor Medicorum.* " His discovery of the circulation had entered the world "with great disadvantages," because it was opposed by "the Grandees of this Profession," who might have stifled this "Infant opinion by their Authority." But truth won out; Harvey lived to see "his *Son* and *Heir,* " the circulation of the blood, "at full age and generally received." His work on generation was "as yet in its minority," but "growing up apace into publick credit." Harvey was a second Linacre and great benefactor to the College of Physicians, which had erected an inscribed statue in his honor. And he might have been an even greater benefactor to all mankind, had not the unhappy dissension of the Civil War destroyed the papers in which Harvey had laid down "a Practice of Physick" conformable to the circulation.[94] Edward Chamberlayne, in his guidebook to English life and institutions, developed the same theme of the benefactor. The "ever famous Dr. Harvey" had erected a magnificent structure at the College to serve as a library and meeting room, and had turned over his "whole Inheritance" to his colleagues, part of which he assigned "for an Anniversary Harangue to commemorate all their Benefactors, to exhort others to follow their good Examples, and to provide a plentiful Dinner for the worthy Company."[95]

As Harvey's name and the factual nature of his discoveries came to be recognized outside strictly medical circles, they took on wider methodological significance. To Thomas Hobbes, writing in *De corpore* (1655), Harvey had not only written wonderfully acute books on the motion of the blood and the generation of animals, he also exemplified how great a man it took to have his discoveries recognized in his own lifetime.[96] For Henry More, Harvey's discovery exemplified how difficult it was to penetrate into our very selves. Had not man's genius deciphered the orbits of the planets long before that venerable Englishman, Harvey, placed before an amazed world the unalterable circuits of man's own purple fluid?[97]

James Harrington and Matthew Wren exchanged political tracts in which *inter alia* they debated the methodological point of whether the principles of politics could be extracted from an individual kind of government, in the same way as Harvey had discovered the circulation by anatomizing bodies. Harrington, writing in 1656 against Hobbes's political views, said Hobbes's logic was "as if a man should tell famous *Hervey*, that he transcribed his *Circulation* of the *bloud*, not out of the *Principles of Nature*, but out of the *Anatomy* of this or that body."[98] In the following year Wren answered Harrington in kind, arguing that simply because *"Hervey* in his Circulation hath followed the principles of nature," did not mean that Harrington could assume the same method was possible in political philosophy.[99] The Harvey image appeared in Harrington's and Wren's mutual ripostes of 1658 and 1659, becoming more complex as it was elaborated, but always retaining Harvey and his circulation as a model deduction from nature.[100] Harrington even used the discovery of the circulation to argue society's need for an innovator, in this case a single legislator to lay down a plan of government:

> *Invention* is a solitary thing. All the Physicians in the world put together invented not the circulation of the bloud, nor can invent any such thing, though in their own Art; yet this was invented by One alone, and being invented is unanimously voted and embraced by the generality of Physicians.[101]

Themes both of methodology and of theology are most interestingly exemplified in the works of one of the most popular of late seventeenth-century English philosophers, Robert Boyle.[102] His cognizance of Harvey's work came early in his career, in the period ca. 1647–1657, when Boyle was in his twenties. During these years Boyle lived in Dorsetshire, London, Oxford, and Dublin, meeting in each of those places disciples of Harvey—such as Highmore, Joyliffe, Clarke, Willis, Bathurst, and Petty—and engaging with them in dissections. Although an aristocrat whose condition enabled him "to make Experiments by others Hands," Boyle had not "been so nice as to decline dissecting *Dogs, Wolves, Fishes,* and even Rats and Mice," with his own hands.[103] He early accepted the circulation,[104] read *De generatione* closely,[105] and met Harvey on several occasions. He visited Harvey at his lodgings, discussed medical cases, and even questioned Harvey about what had led him to the circulation.[106] Thus it is not surprising that in tracts of natural theology written during this decade, in addition to his more properly scientific works, the example of Harvey and his discoveries was adduced on a number of occasions.

For Boyle, anatomy in general and the circulation in particular evidenced the existence and attributes of the divine being. Boyle saw greater enlightenment in "dead and stinking Carkases" than in courts and libraries, for one may trace "in those forsaken Mansions, the inimitable Workmanship of the Omniscient Architect."[107] He that is a stranger to anatomy "shall never be able to discern in the circulation of the blood, the motion of the Chyle, and the contrivance of all the parts of a humane Body, those Proofs, as well as Effects," of the omniscient artificer.[108] Similar edification may be obtained from observing embryonic development. As traced out by Highmore and by "that great promoter of Anatomical Knowledge, Dr. Harvey," nature's exquisite method in the order and fashioning of a chick showed God's providence and goodness.[109] Harvey's explanation of foetal circulation made the same point; blood bypassed the lungs *in utero,* "So careful is Nature not to do things in vain."[110] Indeed, Boyle wrote, when

I study the Book of Nature, and consult the Glosses of Aristotle, Epicurus, Paracelsus, Harvey, Helmont, and other learn'd Expositors of that instructive Volume; I find my self oftentimes reduc'd to exclaim with the Psalmist, *How manifold are thy works, O Lord? in wisdom hast thou made them all* (Psalm 104.24).[111]

Boyle believed that this divinely created harmony of the parts therefore assured us that our frequent dissections would be rewarded with new discoveries, a truth illustrated vividly in the case of Harvey. Before him "many Learned Anatomists," even for "all their diligent contemplation of humane Bodies, never dream'd (for ought appears) of so advantageous an use of the Valves of the Heart, nor that nimble Circular motion of the Blood." In fact, it was consideration of these valves, as he himself told Boyle, that "first hinted the Circulation to our Famous *Harvey.* "[112]

Harvey came, with relative rapidity, to be honored in literary works as one of the greatest of the moderns. In 1652 Charleton ranked him among the few true geniuses of the past century. Not every age, he noted, can "boast the production of a *Copernicus, Gilbert, Galilaeo, Mersennus, Cartesius,* or a *Harvy:* Providence introducing such, as Time doth *New Stars,* single and seldom."[113] Hobbes too compared Harvey with Copernicus and Galileo.[114] In 1661 Abraham Cowley suggested that his proposed experimental college should have a gallery with portraits or statues of "all the inventors of anything useful to Humane Life," including one of the author of "the Circulation of the Blood."[115] Cowley's projected college was never built, but he did add his voice to those praising Harvey by publishing his well-known "Ode" in 1663. In that same year John Dryden published a similar, if rather shorter, laudatory poem addressed to Walter Charleton. Dryden placed his friend in the company of those illustrious Englishmen who were "Among th'*Assertors* of free Reason's claim": of philosophers, Bacon, Gilbert and Boyle; of physicians, Harvey and Ent.[116]

This same theme of Harvey as one of the English leaders of the "Moderns" was elaborated at some length by the Royal Society's self-appointed spokesman, Joseph Glanvill. As a way of defending the Society's enterprise, he chronicled in his *Plus Ultra* (1668) the recent improvements in all the sciences, including anatomy. He recounted almost two dozen new structures discovered by anatomists in the past seventy-five years, including those by such Englishmen as Highmore, Joyliffe, Wharton, Glisson, and Willis.[117]

But of all the *modern Discoveries, Wit* and *Industry* have made in the *Oeconomy* of *humane Nature,* the Noblest is that of the *Circulation* of the *Blood,* which was the Invention of our deservedly-famous *Harvey.*[118]

Moreover, Glanvill wrote, those who would read into the works of Hippocrates, Plato, or Aristotle some knowledge of the circulation, were like the religious enthusiasts who pretended to find the course of political events in the revelations of St. John. Would not such a theory, had the ancients had it, have become well known? Only the imaginings of the envious would ascribe to the ancients the glory and honor of discovery that belongs to Harvey. Some credit may perhaps be due to modern claimants, such as Paulus Venetus, Prosper Alpinus, or Andreas Caesalpinus, but this merely vindicated the moderns all the more.[119] In any case, Glanvill was most concerned "to have *Justice* for that Excellent Man," which, he notes, has now been done:

And the World hath now done *right* to his *Memory, Death* having overcome that *Envy* which *dogs living Virtue* to the *Grave;* and his *Name* rests quietly in the Arms of *Glory,* while the *Pretensions* of his *Rivals* are *creeping* into *darkness* and *oblivion.*[120]

All of these themes, from the simple facts of Harvey's discoveries and their allegorical meanings, to the larger implications of Harvey's discoveries for the controversy over the relative merits of the ancients and moderns, were neatly recapitulated in poems published in 1653 and 1656 by two physicians, Martin Llewellyn and John Collop. The former had an especially close relation to Harvey, having been with him at the Oxford siege, as well as being a member of the College and a friend of Cartwright and Berkenhead.[121]

Harvey's great glory, Llewellyn said, was to overthrow the dictates of "gray *Antiquity,*" and to prove that *"Science* is not *Creed.*"[122] Llewellyn scorned those who respected years rather than truth: "Who for their *Age* alone doe *Writers* trust,/Prize *Armour,* not for th'*Proof,* but for the *Rust.*" He praised Harvey for looking beyond the cant of ancient volumes to nature itself:

> From *Books* to *Nature* thy *Appeale* is made,
> Thy *Copies* by their *Archetype* are swayd.
> Though *High* and *Reverend* thy *Authors* sit,
> Yet the *Creation* is thy *Classick Writ.*[123]

Harvey's cunning knife found truth not just in a "dull Emerit Carcase," "But in the *Living Laboratories,* when/ The *Vitals* ply'd their task like *Lab'ring men.*"[124]

> There thy *Observing* Eye first found the Art
> Of all the *Wheels* and *Clock-work* of the *Heart:*
> The *mystick causes* of its *Dark Estate,*
> What Pullies *Close* its *Cells,* and what *Dilate,*
> What secret Engines tune the *Pulse,* whose din
> By *Chimes without, Strikes* how things fare *within.*[125]

Harvey had traced the crimson blood round its course; like Drake he became a *"Circulator* of the *Lesser World."* Despisers arose at once, and Europe "with hot *combustions* rung." But soon a "swarm of *Champion Pens"* appeared, experience vanquished ancient defense, "And *Prejudice* was captive led by *Sense.*"[126]

John Collop, also an M.D. although no Collegian,[127] traced out similar themes in a book of poems.[128] Many treated medical subjects; no less than six referred to Harvey and his discoveries,[129] including one specifically "On Doctor Harvey." Alluding to the statue, or pillar, of Harvey erected at the College of Physicians, Collop called Harvey "truths pillar too."[130] Harvey was Hercules, cleaning the Augean stables of ancient filth, and using his dissecting knife instead of a club to slay the seven-headed hydra of error. Harvey had set sail on the purple flood of our blood, circled through the microcosm,

and made us understand the world within ourselves. By the cunning of his
knife, he had made the dead yield up the secrets of life. Harvey's accomplishment was his own best monument: "What need we pillars unto *Harvey*
raise,/ Who rears himself a Pyramid of praise?"[131] In this he had the help of
Glisson, and especially of Ent, who was not only "Great Harvey's second," a
herald who proclaimed "our Williams Conquest," but a man who opened
nature's books to men, and taught them to read.[132]

Collop wove into a poem "Of the Blood" all of Harvey's new discoveries.
Blood "doth circle through the lesser world"; it was sun-like, giving motion,
life and sense; although it existed before either the heart or the liver, without
its own innate heat it became nothing but cruor.[133] Both sets of Collop's
themes—Harvey's example and his discoveries—were once again cleverly
combined in yet another poem satirizing a "Piss-pot prophet" who railed
against the College of Physicians:

> I never durst approach the Colledg near,
> They Bishop like do place an Image there.
> Their Idol-*Harvy* of the Serpents breed,
> To break his head denys the woman seed.
> We're wonderfully made the Scripture saies,
> Yet this wretch how we're made would show the waies;
> Nay, Conjurer-like makes Circling in the blood,
> I know not why, but sure it can't be good.
> What spirit 'tis he trades with is unknown
> Distinct from blood he will no spirits own.[134]

Harvey and the Harveians for the Defense of Physicians

Given Harvey's growing fame among both physicians and the London
intelligentsia, it is not surprising that his colleagues invoked his name to dis-
arm critics of the medical profession. Traditional learned medicine in general, and the College of Physicians in particular, were especially subjected to
a barrage of such criticisms in the late 1660s and early 1670s.[135] Helmontians
like Marchamont Nedham proclaimed the bankruptcy of Galenic clinical
concepts and medicaments, and the superiority of chemical remedies.[136] The
insurgents got so far as to found, in early 1665, a Society of Chemical Physicians as a rival to the College.[137] Apothecaries, physicians believed, practiced
medicine with increasing boldness, a menace some proposed to counter by
compounding their own prescriptions. Such issues were mooted with great

vehemence in the pamphlet war that ensued, with Harvey figuring in almost all of the physicians' responses—and sometimes in the attacks as well.

Harvey was regularly cited as *princeps* in the list of anatomists whose brilliant discoveries justified the corporate existence of the College of Physicians. Merrett (1665) believed that the learned members of the College had "advanc'd Physick more these last forty years, than any one Society of Physicians in Europe," and would continue to do so, such that "as our Nation has had the honour of one of the best things that ever was discover'd in the Theory of Physick, The Bloods Circulation; so it may give an example to all the world of the best, and soundest, and most rational way of Practice."[138] Nathaniel Hodges (1665) was more specific; he could "confidently affirm, that the most *considerable discoveries* which in these later *Ages* have merited *applause* and *credit* in the World, were most happily *made* by some *Members* of this *Society,* witness the *Renowned Doctor* Harvey's *circulation of the Blood, Doctor* Jolive's *first observation of the Lymphaeducts,* and many others."[139] Timothy Clarke (1670) extended the list yet again, and tied it directly to Harvey. He asserted that "since the time that *our great Doctor Harvey* acquired that honour to himself, and to our nation in his excellent Anatomical discoveries, our younger physicians"—he cited especially Glisson, Wharton, and Ent—"grew generously to emulate both his fortune, and endeavours, and perhaps the World hath not a Society of our profession, in which considering the number of them, there are so many excellent Anatomists."[140] Clarke detailed the activities of the research committees of the College, noted that all of this was done without publicly supported physic-gardens, laboratories, or endowed professors save in anatomy, and proudly concluded that the College "hath more advanced the true knowledg of Physick, within this last forty years, than any one Society of Physitians in Europe."[141]

The Helmontians accused Collegians of being blindly loyal to the ancients. Exactly the opposite was true, physicians retorted. Harvey and his followers had led the moderns in discovery, thereby mending ancient doctrines. Robert Sprackling (1665), although he defended the clinical insights of Hippocrates, acknowledged that "the late eminent discoveries have in many things corrected the unanimous errings of Antiquity, and in other things produced de novo doctrines of singular use and importance." Who, he queried, "can compare the Treatise of *Hippocrates Peri kardies* to that of Doctor *Harvey de motu Cordis,* or the one *Peri gonis* to the other *De Generatione?*" The works of Glisson, Ent, and Wharton similarly surpassed their Hippocratean predecessors.[142] George Castle (1667) believed that "since the Circulation of the Blood has been found out by Doctor Harvey," medicine had been laid upon a new foundation, and "the whole Fabrick has been built from the very ground."[143]

This had been carried out, physicians said, not by empirics and self-styled chemists pretending to experiment, but by learned men. In their polemics the physicians used the example of Harvey and his followers to emphasize the close links that bound together medical education, experimental inquiry, and anatomical innovation. Clarke ranked Harvey, Glisson and Ent with the revered Bacon and Gilbert, and asserted that "few men are so well qualified" to promote the experimental way of knowledge "as well educated physicians."[144] To prove his point that learned men, not empirics, were responsible for the "vaste improvement of Physick," Castle had only to list their names: Harvey, Glisson, Ent, Highmore, Wharton and Willis.[145] Daniel Cox felt that learned physicians, educated first as natural philosophers, acquired thereby an inclination toward experiment and observation, which in turn gave rise to

...those Noble productions of their Brains, which will perpetuate their Names, and oblige all Mankind that shall succeed them. Of how great use was that admirable invention of *Harvie's* concerning the Blood's Circulation? and, What great advantages may we derive from the Inventions of *Pecquet, Glisson, Ent, Wharton, Bartholine, Willis, Needham, Lower,* and other excellent Anatomists?[146]

The physicians' training and professional status enabled them to employ their unmatched talents in "Physiological Researches" and *"Anatomical experiments"* that eventually would disclose "knowledge of the true and natural uses of each part."[147]

Some Helmontians, such as Marchamont Nedham, had seemed to deprecate the importance of anatomy;[148] Collegiate physicians leapt to its defense. Sprackling was amazed that Nedham should say that anatomy was useless, when it was the very basis of surgery, diagnosis and therapy.[149] A competent knowledge of anatomy, John Twysden (1666) said, is necessary for the cure of diseases.[150] Far from being useless, "he that shall read *Harvey's* works, Dr. *Glissons* book *de anat. hepatis,* Dr. *Wharton de glandulis, Pécket de vasis chiliferis,* and others, will find how much the world is beholding to them for their pains therein, and the Art enriched by their discoveries."[151] Just as navigation depended on astronomy, and surveying on geometry, so did medicine depend on anatomy: "the curious and useful speculations of some few, are able to give a competent stock of knowledge to all others, without wholly taking them off from their more necessary employment in the cure of diseases."[152] Castle said in praise of anatomy that "Dogs, Pigs and Monkeys, have contributed more to the advancement of Physick than [Marchamont Nedham] and his fraternity ever did, or are like to do."[153]

Harvey entered the fray in ways other than as the archetypal anatomist. In one pamphlet Christopher Merrett, the Harveian Librarian, appealed to the memory of his mentor when he answered sarcastically Henry Stubbe's insulting inquiries as to his qualifications: "the immortal Dr. Harvey was to blame in nominating with some Eulogy such a pitiful Physician to be his Library keeper, who necessarily was to converse with learned forreiners and travailers in the Art of Physic."[154] Indeed, Merrett thought it "no disrepute to be detracted from" by Stubbe, who had "endeavoured to diminish my most honoured friends, the ever renowned Dr. Harvey, Mr. Boyl, Dr. Willis, Dr. Lower," and "many other famous men of our Nation."[155]

One of the more interesting exchanges of ink on Harveian themes occurred between Nedham and Twysden. Nedham, although slighting the applicability of anatomy to medicine, had praised such modern anatomists as Glisson, Highmore, Willis, and "the immortal *Harvey.*"[156] He even used Harvey to make a few of his points against the Galenists. In one passage Nedham cited Harvey, along with Helmont, Descartes, and others, as examples of men who had been persecuted by their colleagues for having doubted the ancient philosophers and physicians.[157] In another, Nedham criticized Hippocrates for believing in "the four fancies called Humours," and said that "our Hippocrates (as some call him) Dr *Harvey* approves not, and allows but one."[158]

Such misrepresentations of the great physician incensed Harvey's friend and kinsman, John Twysden.[159] He retorted that Nedham would have us overthrow all, merely on his own authority.[160] Besides, had not Nedham himself lived to see such innovators honored, and their truths embraced?

Who is more famous or esteemed all the world over, than the most learned Dr. *Harvey,* whose statue set up in the publike College, and Anniversary Oration upon his account will preserve his memory perhaps longer than the numerous more noble progeny deduced from other branches of that ancient and deserving family, whose notions have been more improved, and whose writings in their kind more admired?[161]

Moreover, said Twysden, Nedham misread the modern Hippocrates in criticizing the ancient one. Twysden analyzed the passages in *De generatione* to which Nedham had referred, and proved that they did not deny the four humors.[162] On the contrary, Harvey admired the ancients, especially Aristotle. Twysden had had, he said, "the honor to know him many years," and

Harvey had often said that Aristotle was "the most rational and acute Philosopher that ever lived."[163] Twysden would clearly not stand idly by and see the Harveian myth serve the opponents of learned medicine.

The anatomical defense of learned medicine, utilizing the accomplishments of Harvey and his successors, reached its height in the historico-polemical works of Charles Goodall.[164] Almost a quarter of his first book, *The College of Physicians Vindicated* (1676), was devoted to the relationship between anatomy and medicine.[165] Had not "all the diagnosticks of physick and methods of cure in all Ages" been "derived out of Anatomy?" Thus Harvey had devoted much time to anatomical studies, and to his books on the circulation and on generation. In this he had been followed by Glisson, Wharton, Willis, Walter Needham, and Lower.[166] Goodall argued with many examples that a knowledge of anatomy made for better therapy.[167] He enlarged at even greater length on the argument that it was the moderns who had most improved the anatomic part of medicine.[168] This had its beginning in Harvey. One could not overestimate the benefit he had "done to the publick by that surprizing and admirable discovery of the circulation of the blood, which hath since been universally embraced and given him so great a name through out the world."[169] Harvey had been followed in turn by a line of great successors, each of whom had illuminated his own particular part of medicine: Glisson on the liver, sanguification and the bile; Willis on the animal spirits and the anatomical loci of convulsive diseases; Wharton on the glands and saliva; Ent on the circulation and the *succus nervosus;* Needham on the chyle and saliva, and velocity of circulation.[170] Finally, Goodall took the battle into the enemy camp by arguing that in recent times—witness men like Willis—the greatest anatomists and practitioners had also been well versed in chemistry.[171]

Goodall took a slightly different tack in his second polemical work, *The Royal College of Physicians of London Founded and Established by Law* (1684). In the midst of inundating the reader with documents proving the legal rights of the College to regulate practice, he devoted almost sixty pages to biographical sketches of the College's most illustrious members.[172] The longest, most naturally, was of Harvey.[173] Goodall emphasized how Harvey had read *De motu cordis* to the College as his Lumleian Lectures, and rejected, citing Charleton and Borelli, the rival claims of priority in the discovery of the circulation. He quoted at length from Ent's preface to *De generatione,* emphasizing Harvey's retiring nature, his unflagging zeal for dissection, his desire to go beyond Aristotle and Galen, his modesty in bringing out his studies of generation, and the ease with which discovery, though purchased by much effort, came to him. Goodall summarized in some detail the contents of *De motu cordis* and *De generatione,* and gave a detailed list of the treatises that had perished. He closed by eulogizing Harvey's benefactions to the College, and reproducing the long and fulsome memorial inscription engraved under Harvey's portrait at the College.

Harvey's successors came in for a similar, if briefer, treatment: Glisson, Willis, Ent, Scarburgh, Charleton, Lower, and Needham—all had their lives sketched, their publications noted, and their contributions to anatomy and to medicine enumerated in some detail.[174] The overall effect, if rather ponderous, is nonetheless impressive. One sees Harvey, not merely as a scientist and philanthropist, but hypostatized into the raison d'être of the College, the founder of a powerful new anatomical and investigative concept of a physician.

Attacks on the Harveian Myth: Henry Stubbe and Gideon Harvey

It would be too much to expect of human nature that every writer should be content to speak *de mortuis nil nisi bonum;* some authors did disparage Harvey in particular, and the tradition of the anatomical physician for which he had come to stand. In each case it seems clear that they bore Harvey no animus personally, but were merely reacting in kind to the growing use of Harvey's name to justify what they felt was not justifiable.

In his *Plus Ultra* (1668) Joseph Glanvill had used Harvey's accomplishments, among other pieces of evidence, to uphold the moderns against the ancients.[175] Glanvill's fellow Oxonian Henry Stubbe, a Warwick physician and sometime member of Oxford scientific circles, could not abide such literary license. Although professedly an admirer of the College of Physicians, his pedant's instincts were aroused sufficiently by what he saw as Glanvill's overstatements to attempt to prove that Harvey was not as much the innovator as commonly conceived. In his *Plus Ultra Reduced to a Non Plus* (1670), Stubbe set out inter alia to examine "The *Original* and *Progress of Anatomy*" and the question of "The *First Inventor* of the *Circulation of the Blood.*"[176]

On the question of anatomical innovation, Stubbe praised the investigations of the ancients, especially the dissections of Aristotle and the great dexterity and discoveries of Galen.[177] True, they had occasionally erred, but had not Harvey, Highmore, and other moderns also made mistakes?[178] Besides, Harvey himself was known to have praised Aristotle frequently for his

penetrating inquisitiveness into all parts of nature.[179] Even among those
discoveries admittedly of recent times, Stubbe said, Glanvill was mistaken in
assigning priority. Realdo Colombo had long ago demonstrated the circulation of the blood through the lungs. The venous valves were discovered "by
Paul, the Venetian Monk," who had shown them to Fabricius. The anatomical discoveries attributed by Glanvill to Willis were largely Lower's doing.
And Glisson's discovery of a nutritious juice distributed by the nerves was far
from being accepted by all physicians.[180]

But for Stubbe the most debatable point of priority concerned the
discovery of the circulation. Numerous moderns—many of them admirers of
Harvey—had allowed that there were many passages in the ancients that
seemed to hint of their knowledge of the circulation. Stubbe believed that if
one examined the appropriate passages from Hippocrates, Plato, and Aristotle, one would see that although *"all men* do give unto *Harvey* the credit of
having so explicated it, and *Anatomically* proved" the circulation, he built
on his predecessors in the same way as Epicurus had developed the atomism
of Democritus and Leucippus.

Nor hath *Harvey* any other *Plea* and *Right* to the *Invention,* then that *he* did more
fully and *perspicuously* declare *it,* and in the most *judicious* and *solid* manner assert
what others had but *hinted* at, or *faintly* insisted on.[181]

Even among the moderns, Stubbe said, there were several claimants whose
work should be examined, most especially Andreas Caesalpinus.[182] Stubbe
then proceeded, step by step, to recapitulate the Harveian view of the heart,
its vessels, the lungs, the blood, the pulse, the pulmonary circulation, the
arterial outflow and venous return—in each case giving quotes and
references to Caesalpinus's *Quaestionum peripateticarum* (1571) and
Questionum medicarum (1593) to prove that the Tuscan had anticipated
Harvey.[183] Just as important for Stubbe's argument, Caesalpinus was a strict
and passionate follower of Aristotle. Stubbe summed up:

I have demonstrated that *Andraeas Caesalpinus,* a rigid *Peripatetick* upon *sensible
Experiments & Mechanical considerations,* not *notional apprehensions,* did not only
discover this *motion* of the blood (even *through the Lungs*) but gave it the name of
CIRCULATIO SANGUINIS.[184]

Indeed, Stubbe said, it seemed likely that Harvey, "who was a *Peripatetique*
Physician" trained at Padua among the greatest Aristotelian anatomists and
philosophers, "did take up this opinion from *my Author.*"[185] This interpreta-

tion was made more probable, Stubbe said, by Harvey's failure to assert, in any of his books, that he was truly the discoverer of the circulation.

He no where asserts the *Invention* so to *himself*, as to deny that he had the *intimation* or *notion* from *Caesalpinus;* but leaves the *Controversy* in the dark: which *silence* of his I take for a *tacite Confession.* His *Ambition* of *Glory* made him willing to be thought the *Authour* of a *Paradox* he had so illustrated, and *brought upon the Stage,* when it lay *unregarded,* and in all probability *buried in oblivion.* Yet such was his *Modesty,* as not to vindicate it to *himself* by telling a *Lie.* And such his *Prudence,* as rather to avoid the *debate,* then resolve it to *his prejudice.* [186]

Having so disparaged him, Stubbe generously conceded that Harvey "had *parts* and *industry* enough to have *discovered* it, had he not been *prevented therein.* "[187]

Nor was the circulation itself the great invention some would have it to be. Many questions were still left unresolved. How did the blood pass through the lungs? What was the cause of the heart's pulsation? Was blood diffused throughout the body, or did it remain within vessels? Was there any difference between arterial and venous blood? How did the circulation affect phlebotomy and the doctrine of the pulse?[188] Even if these questions should be answered, the circulation had not overthrown *"the usual methods of Physick,"* nor introduced *"new* and *beneficial* discoveries in that part of Medicine which is Therapeutick." Indeed, Harvey himself denied that it would change the medicine handed down from the ancients.[189]

Given such a broad attack on Harvey's originality and probity, it is not surprising that when Glanvill in turn rebutted Stubbe, he also spoke about Harvey.[190] Since Glanvill was no physician, and rather less of a scholar than Stubbe, he wisely chose not to trade learned references. He had, Glanvill said, already noted such claimants as Caesalpinus, but concluded that "almost all men" now "ascribe the *Invention* to D. *Harvy.* "[191] Glanvill reiterated that both men served equally well his purpose of demonstrating the superiority of the moderns over the ancients.[192] As for Stubbe's assertion that Harvey nowhere claimed to have discovered the circulation, this only showed Stubbe's ignorance of Harvey's works. Glanvill then quoted Harvey from *De generatione* that "the admirable circulation of the blood originally discovered by me, I have lived to see admitted by almost all."[193]

Another Harvey detractor, William's namesake Gideon, was motivated not so much by pique and pendantry gone astray, but by vitriolic outrage at physicians who used anatomical accomplishments to advance their professional careers. In books published in the early 1670s this London physician,

although not a member of the College of Physicians, expressed admiration
for it[194] and for the anatomical accomplishments of its Fellows. Just as Hippocrates had laid one basis for medicine on the island of Cos, so had a
modern Hippocrates, "Doctor *William Harvey,* of Immortal Memory," laid
a new foundation for medicine "by Detecting the *Circulation of the Blood,*
for which this *Britain* may as justly Merit the Title of *Divine,* as the other
Cous."[195] He praised Ent for his defense of the circulation, Wharton for his
work on glands and ducts, Glisson for his discoveries about the liver, Glisson
with his colleagues for their work concerning rickets, and lauded Willis
although disagreeing with some of his ideas about the blood.[196] His only passing objection was to a physician—he meant here Richard Lower—who "hath
but once or twice dissected a Sheeps-head, or a Calves-pluck," and thereby
thought himself an "expert Anatomist," able to contradict his colleagues.[197]
Gideon Harvey had obviously had a run-in with Lower.

Their paths crossed again in 1676, when both treated an injured noble-
man.[198] Gideon Harvey was so incensed by the way Lower dominated the case
that he published a tract[199] denouncing this "Anatomical Physician," who by
virtue of his College membership, his association with Willis, and his ability
to impress novices by flaying a few dogs or cats, "engrosses all."[200]

Harvey's sense of outrage continued to fester until, in 1683, he published *The Conclave of Physicians,*[201] a blistering attack on the College of
Physicians, many of its members, its anatomical research, "the specious and
false pretensions of Anatomical Physitians," the uselessness of anatomy, or
rather its false usefulness in promoting the careers of physicians whose
clinical skills were negligible. The College assembled often in winter, Harvey
said, to celebrate their "immolations" upon dogs, cats, "and sometimes
upon humane bodies." But what had come of all this in twenty years? Almost
nothing.[202] Physicians dwelt upon this "introductory part of Physick," and
"seldom or never" arrived at a considerable proficiency in the art of
medicine.[203] In fact, "those pretended Anatomical Physitians, who have so
belabour'd and tortur'd the particular parts, are generally the least knowing
in the whole body of Anatomy."[204] Such a man was nothing but "a Dog-
fleyer" who "scribl'd a Treatise of the Heart, Lungs, Brains, Womb, or
some other Entrails (though of no use)," and belonged to a College that was
nothing but "a Herd of learned Quacks, Renegado-Divines, School-masters,
Apothecaries and Barbers, a rare Hodge-pot of Physicians."[205] The illusion
of research was created to attract customers, Gideon believed; Willis's Oxford practice "was so inconsiderable, that he was forced to block at his Pen,
and so by forging of Novelties," attract patients.[206]

Gideon Harvey followed exactly the same line in attacking his very namesake a few years later. He used William Harvey to exemplify how "needless curiosities, and too fine spun Speculations of Anatomy," profited the physician not at all.[207] Harvey, "the greatest Anatomist of his time, and no extraordinary Physician,"[208] erred glaringly in prescribing for squire Rainton of Enfield. In another case Harvey mistook a tumor for an aneurism. Gideon further detailed how Harvey's mismanagement of the cases stemmed from hubris based upon his anatomical pretensions.[209] In another case recounted by Gideon, a patient with sciatica refused Harvey's expensive and anatomically-based treatment, and was cured by another physician who, although no anatomist, was gifted with the sagacity to know diseases when presented to him.[210]

In this particular exchange the anatomical physicians once again had the last word. Thomas Guidott answered Gideon Harvey a year later in a marvelous mock-heroic poem of doggerel couplets.[211] Guidott played upon the identical names in castigating Gideon for aspersions cast on William:

> But can that *Name*, fam'd for *Bloods Circulation*
> Turn *Holocaust* to Spleen, and Emulation?
> Bold *Heterodox*, of prostituted Fame!
> Cease to be *Physicks-Zoil*, or change they Name,
> Degenerate *Mome*, born to confute that *Thame*
> None of *Great Harvey's* Blood *circles* in him.[212]

Guidott went on to praise Willis at great length, and to recount and extol the anatomical discoveries about the muscles, arteries, brain, lacteals, and ducts that Gideon had seen as so useless.[213] Most of all Guidott praised the circulation, the embodiment of anatomy's triumph:

> The famed *Circle* that the blood doth make,
> The *Circuit* it do's round the body take,
> A *Circuit* that is but a Visitation,
> To help each part, and keep it in its station,
> Discoverd by *a man*, whose very name
> To haters of Anatomy's a shame,
> We justly owe to his *Industrious art*,
> Declares the blood comes from, flows to the *Heart*.[214]

The Emergence and Nature of the Harveian Myth

The rapidity with which Harvey and his accomplishments grew to symbolic status is particularly striking. There was almost no popular or literary perception of him in the 1640s; it emerged gradually in the 1650s, and had become quite strong by the 1660s. The evidence suggests some reasons why. The circular motion of the blood, once it had gained the imprimatur of the anatomists, was a concept at once sufficiently simple and sufficiently vivid to make Harvey's achievement easily comprehensible. It was a unit idea, statable in a sentence. It could thus be assimilated either as a single datum by the less educated, or in a more complex form by those who had encountered it at the university. Blood had always had a rich and complex imagery; that it was now set into perpetual motion only increased its evocative qualities. Thus the references in poems, theological tracts, and philosophical works: they betokened as much as they caused a man's rise to public reputation. Litterateurs like Hobbes, More, Harrington, Birkenhead, Cowley, Dryden, and Fuller would not have dropped Harvey references into their works if they had not had reasons to feel that the literate public had some vague understanding of his accomplishments.

It is interesting in this respect to compare the popular recognition of Harvey's two major works, *De motu cordis* and *De generatione*. While there were many general references to the fact of the circulation, these seldom, with the exception of More, showed any detailed knowledge of *De motu cordis* and the specific arguments it made. By the 1650s, when the Harvey myth began to build, such recourse to the original was unnecessary because a number of anatomical textbooks used in the universities presented the circulation, not as an idea to be debated, but as an accepted physiological fact. Conversely, *De generatione,* a treatise relatively neglected by modern scholars, seems to have exercised a great influence in its own right, and to have contributed significantly to Harvey's reputation. It was available both in Latin and English, and seems to have been widely read even beyond medical circles.

The Harvey myth clearly emerged from acquaintance and friendship. Especially in the 1650s and early 1660s, many of those who saw in his accomplishments something beyond limited anatomical discoveries were likewise his friends. Merrett, Greaves, Scarburgh, Charleton, Llewellyn, Berkenhead, Hobbes, More, Cowley, Boyle and Twysden—all had personal contacts with Harvey of varying degrees of intimacy. It was along these lines of personal relationship that Harvey's reputation, and interpretations of his discoveries, radiated to the world outside anatomy proper.

Perhaps more importantly, as almost all the commentators agree, the Harvey symbol grew because he had not just friends and followers, but successors—men like Glisson, Ent, Wharton, Willis, and later Needham and Lower—who were seen as carrying on his investigatory tradition. That only some of them actually worked in the areas he pioneered was beside the point; they were clearly active, productive anatomists. It was very much easier to praise a great man if you thereby also praised your colleagues. That past was especially important which extended into the present.

These successors were in turn related to another characteristic of the emergence of the Harvey myth—its institutional base in the College of Physicians. Harvey's statue, the Harveian Museum and Library, were physical reminders of the nature and content of Harvey's accomplishments, a presence ritually recalled every year in the Harveian Oration. The relationship was symbiotic; the College spread Harvey's fame, and then in turn invoked that fame to defend its character and corporate privileges.

Politics, of several kinds, also clearly played a part in the establishment of Harvey's reputation. His connection with Charles I, which had been a source of discomfort for Harvey in the late 1640s and early 1650s, became an advantage in the rising tide of monarchical fervor that carried Charles's son back into power. Medical politics in the 1660s, 1670s, and 1680s caused Harvey's repute to be even more assiduously cultivated in succeeding years.

In the course of Harvey's rise to symbolic status in Commonwealth and Restoration England, he and his accomplishments came to be portrayed in a number of recurring images of a professional, methodological, and even theological and historical character.

Professionally, Harvey was the model of the anatomical physician. The learned doctor had traditionally commanded respect because of his knowledge of, and access to, the wisdom of the Hippocratic and Galenic works. By the mid-seventeenth century, that societal respect was no longer forthcoming. Harvey's scientific accomplishments, and those of his perceived successors, both originated and validated a new self-image for English, and especially, London, physicians. This was particularly appropriate, because it was in part Harvey's discoveries that had cast the older definition of a physician into disrepute. This new model was particularly congenial because Harvey was not only a man of (almost) unimpeachable anatomical accomplishments, but also one known to be learned in, and deeply respectful of, the ancients. Moreover, training in anatomy and contributions to its advancement were exactly those qualifications which set regular physicians apart from self-styled chemists and empirics. Collegians therefore emphasized the importance to medicine of anatomy and new anatomical discoveries such as those of Harvey, while their opponents were forced either to denigrate the medical significance of anatomy or, as in the case of the Helmontian George Thomson, to claim anatomical innovations of their own.

Harvey's work was seen, almost from the very beginning, as having methodological significance. Harvey himself had begun this interpretative tradition by insisting prominently in all his works that he professed to learn, "not from books but from dissections, not from the tenets of Philosophers but from the fabric of Nature." Harvey's admirers, from Llewellyn and Colop to Goodall, rang changes on this theme. Harvey, they agreed, had revolutionized medical science not by words and disputation, but by observation, dissection, and vivisection—by direct appeal to sense experience. Medical polemicists emphasized these aspects especially in countering the charges of chemical physicians, one of whose major threats was that they laid claim to their own unique source of sense experience.

When Harvey's work was seen to have theological significance, it was because he exemplified how original investigation displayed to best advantage the wisdom of God manifested in the works of creation. His discoveries in physiology and embryology, as Boyle and later natural theologians discovered, beautifully exemplified the Aristotelian maxim (of which Harvey approved and was often accused of denying) that nature did nothing in vain.

Finally, Harvey and his work were seen as having a kind of historical-ideological significance. He rapidly assumed his place in the elite pantheon of sixteenth and seventeenth-century philosophers and scientists whose accomplishments validated the idea of intellectual progress. In a certain sense, Harvey's presence there served the purpose of the moderns better than that of a Bacon, Descartes, or Mersenne. Harvey's discovery of the circulation shared with those of Copernicus and Galileo a rigor that made it irrefutable, and had the notable advantage of being at once more proximate and concrete than astronomy. Harvey as modern could additionally serve another purpose for an English polemicist: he could be ranked with Gilbert and Bacon to form a triumvirate that made England the intellectual equal of France or Italy.

Allow me to close with a few words of filial piety. I have used such terms as "image," "symbol," and "myth" to characterize the growth of Harvey's reputation. To do so is not, I would argue, to debase the man or his accomplishments. Rather, such an historical analysis reveals those dimensions of perception, pride, and motivation that are as much a part of the practice of science as instruments, experiments, and concepts.

Notes

1. Abraham Cowley, *Verses, Written upon Several Occasions* (London, 1663), pp. 18–21.
2. For a synopsis of these changes in English medicine from the 1540s to the 1620s, see my paper, "The institutional Renaissance of English medicine," forthcoming in *Med. Hist.*

THE IMAGE OF HARVEY   137

3. For details on these changes, see my paper, "The physician as virtuoso in seventeenth-century England" (to be published by the William Andrews Clarke Library, Los Angeles), and the sources therein cited.

4. John Aubrey, *Brief Lives,* ed. Andrew Clark (Oxford: Clarendon Press, 1898), I, 300.

5. See for example, the *Dictionary of National Biography* and William Munk, *The Roll of the Royal College of Physicians of London,* 2nd ed. (London: Longman, 1878), I, 219; Glisson's biography is clarified in R. Milnes Walker, "Francis Glisson and his capsule," *Annals of the Royal College of Surgeons of England,* 1966, *38:*71-91.

6. British Library, MSS. Sloane 574B, 681, 1116, 2251, 2326, 3258, and 3306-15.

7. Ibid., MSS. Sloane 3307, ff. 69-79; 3309, ff. 141-44, 201-4; 3310, f. 369.

8. Ibid., respectively MSS. Sloane 3310, ff. 327, 393-96; 3307, ff. 74-79; 3309, ff. 18-20; 3309, ff. 141-44; 3312, ff. 2-16, 106-28.

9. Ibid., respectively MSS. Sloane 3308, f. 296; 3308, f. 167; 3312, ff. 42-47; 3309, ff. 139-40.

10. [Autobiography of John Wallis], p. cl, in Thomas Hearne (ed.), *Peter Langtoft's Chronicle,* vol. I (Oxford, 1725).

11. British Library, MS. Sloane 3312, ff. 265-68.

12. Ibid., MS. Sloane 3310, ff. 249-55.

13. Ibid., MS. Sloane 3310, f. 301.

14. Ibid., MS. Sloane 3308, ff. 278-81.

15. On Henry Power, see Charles Webster, "Henry Power's experimental philosophy," *Ambix,* 1967, *14:* 150-78.

16. Thomas Browne to Henry Power, [1646]; Power to Browne, 15 September 1648 and 28 August 1649, in *The Works of Sir Thomas Browne,* ed. Geoffrey Keynes (Chicago: University of Chicago Press, 1964), IV, 257, 260, 261-63.

17. F. J. Cole, "Henry Power on the circulation of the blood," *J. Hist., Med.,* 1957, *12:* 291-324.

18. Ibid., p. 294.

19. Lord Edmund Fitzmaurice, *The Life of Sir William Petty* (London: John Murray, 1895), pp. 5-10.

20. John Wallis, *A Defence of the Royal Society* (London, 1678), p. 8.

21. Anthony Wood, *Fasti Oxoniensis,* ed. Philip Bliss (London, 1820), II, 156; Richard Watkins, *Newes from the Dead* (Oxford, 1651), pp. 2-6; *Registrum Convocationis* (1647-1659), pp. 124-25, University of Oxford Archives.

22. These and other medical manuscripts by Petty comprise Volume III of the Petty Papers at Bowood, Calne, Wiltshire. I am indebted to the Marquis of Lansdowne for his kind permission to inspect these manuscripts.

23. Ibid., No. 26.

24. Ibid., No. 4.

25. *Registrum Congregationis* (1634-1647), University of Oxford Archives, ff. 197v, 181r.

26. *Registrum Congregationis* (1648-1659), University of Oxford Archives, f. 150v; the text of this and other of Bathurst's disputations are in Thomas Wharton, *The Life and Literary Remains of Ralph Bathurst, M.D.* (London, 1761), pp. 210-38.

27. *Registrum Congregationis* (1648-1657), f. 150v.

28. Ibid., f. 151v.

29. Ibid., ff. 152v, 153v, 154r; *Registrum Congregationis* (1659-1669), f. 175r.

30. John Ward, MS. "Diary," vol. IX, f. 76v, Folger Shakespeare Library, Washington, D.C.; for a description of these MSS. see my article, "The John Ward diaries: Mirror of seventeenth-century science and medicine," *J. Hist. Med.,* 1974, *29:* 147-79.

31. Geoffrey Keynes, *The Life of William Harvey* (Oxford: Clarendon Press, 1966), p. 270.

32. Johannes Vesling, *Syntagma anatomicum* (Padua, 1651), pp. 117-21.

33. Ibid., p. 121.

34. John Webster, *Academiarum Examen, or the Examination of Academies* (London, 1654), p. 74. Seth Ward, *Vindiciae Academiarum* (Oxford, 1654), pp. 35-36. On the general controversy, see Allen G. Debus, *Science and Education in the Seventeenth Century: The Webster-Ward Debate* (London: Macdonald, 1970), pp. 33-64.

35. Richard Davis, *Catalogus* (London, 1686), Part I, pp. 98, 108-12, 118, 120, 122; (Oxford, 1686), Part II, pp. 78, 83, 89-90, 92.

36. Catalogue of the Richard Allestree Library, Christ Church, Oxford.

37. *Bibliotheca Oweniana* (London, 1684), p. 31.

38. Bathurst's copy of *De generatione* is now in the Radcliffe Science Library, Oxford.

39. John Harrison and Peter Laslett, *The Library of John Locke* (Oxford: Oxford Bibliographical Society, 1965), p. 151. The *De generatione* is marked with a paraph Locke reserved for highly prized works.

40. "Library Catalogue of Henry Stubbe," British Library MS. Sloane 35, f. 17r.

41. *Bibliotheca Levinziana* (London, 1698), p. 34.

42. British Library MS. Egerton 1632, f. 51r.

43. Cf. Keynes, *Harvey,* pp. 77, 111, 148-53, 187-96, 203-5, 216-19, 263-69, 277-84; Webster, "Harvey and the crisis of medicine," pp. 1-12 above.

44. Aubrey, *Brief Lives,* I, 300.

45. William Harvey, *Exercitatio anatomica de motu cordis et sanguinis in animalibus* (Frankfurt, 1628), p. 6.

46. See Allen G. Debus, "Robert Fludd and the circulation of the blood," *J. Hist. Med.,* 1961, *16:* 374-93.

47. James Primrose, *Exercitationes et animadversiones in librum de motu cordis et circulatione sanguinis. Adversus G.Harveum*(London, 1630).

48. Munk, *Roll,* pp. 219, 224; British Library, MS. Sloane 3315, f. 1r.

49. Keynes, *Harvey,* p. 282; Roger Drake, *Vindiciae contra animadversiones D.D. Primirosii* (London, 1641).

50. I have been able to find no evidence of Harvey's attendance in the College Annals, nor is any given in Keynes, *Harvey,* pp. 284-396.

51. George Ent, in William Harvey, *Exercitationes de generatione animalium* (London, 1651), sig. A3r-v.

52. Keynes, *Harvey,* pp. 314-17, 372-73.

53. Lindsay Sharp, "The Royal College of Physicians and interregnum politics," *Med. Hist.,* 1975, *19:* 107-29.

54. Keynes, *Harvey,* p. 297.

55. Ibid., p. 377.

56. Ibid., pp. 381-406.

57. *Biographia Britannica* (London, 1747-66), IV, 2216.

58. Baldwin Hamey, "Praelectiones anatomicae," 1647/8, MS. 143, Royal College of Physicians, London; Richard Catcher, "Lectures on the pathology and anatomy of the human frame before the College of Physicians," British Library MS. Sloane 95, ff. 1-97, 218-64.

59. Keynes, *Harvey,* p. 400; British Library, MS. Sloane 3315, f. 23; Anthony Wood, *Athenae Oxoniensis* (London, 1813-1820), III, 351; Munk, *Roll,* p. 258.

60. Royal College of Physicians, Annals, IV, f. 35a.

61. Aubrey, *Brief Lives,* p. 297.

62. Annals, IV, f. 50a.

63. Keynes, *Harvey,* p. 461.

64. Christopher Merrett, *Catalogus librorum, instrumentorum chirurgicorum, rerum curiosarum, exoticarumque Coll. Med. Lond. quae habentur in Musaeo Harveano* (London, 1660).

65. Ibid., pp. 1, 3, 13-18.

66. Ibid., p. 12.

67. Ibid., pp. 22, 39-40.

68. Ibid., pp. 41-43.

69. Aubrey, *Brief Lives,* pp. 296-97.

70. Annals, IV, f. 53b-54a.

71. Annals, IV, f. 63a.

72. Royal College of Physicians, London, MS. 109.

73. Edward Greaves, *Oratio habita in aedibus Collegii Medicorum Londinensium, 25 Jul. 1661. Die Harvaei memoriae dicato.* (London, 1667), pp. 13-23.

74. Ibid., p. 19.

75. L.M. Payne discovered, identified, and explicated this Oration: "Sir Charles Scarburgh's Harveian Oration, 1662," *J. Hist. Med.,* 1957, *12:* 158-64.

76. Ibid., pp. 162-64.

77. "A New-years-gift to Brian Lord Bishop of Sarum, upon the Author's entring into holy Orders, 1638," in William Cartwright, *Comedies, Tragi-Comedies, With other Poems* (London, 1651), pp. 284-86. This was first noticed by C.A.R. Boyd and S.A.C. Boyd, "An early reference in English poetry to the circulation of the blood," *J. Hist. Med.,* 1970, *25:* 212-14.

78. John Berkenhead, "In Memory of Mr William Cartwright," sig. *8r-[11r] in Cartwright, *Comedies, Tragi-Comedies;* the Harvey reference is on sig. *9r. It was first noticed by Richard A. Hunter and Ida Macalpine, "Sir John Berkenhead's lines on William Harvey, 1651," *J. Hist. Med.,* 1962. *17:* 403-5.

79. F[rancis] V[ernon], *Detur Pulchriori: Or, A Poem in the Praise of the University of Oxford* (Oxford, 1658), p. 3.

80. Thomas Sprat, The Plague of Athens (London, 1659), p. 9.

81. On Charleton generally, see the excellent article by Lindsay Sharp, "Walter Charlton's early life 1620-1659, and relationship to natural philosophy in mid-seventeenth century England," *Ann. Sci.,* 1973, *30:* 311-40.

82. Walter Charleton, *The Darknes of Atheism Dispelled by the Light of Nature. A Physico-Theologicall Treatise* (London, 1652), p. 131.

83. Ibid., p. 295.

84. Walter Charleton, *The Immortality of the Human Soul, Demonstrated by the Light of Nature. In Two Dialogues* (London, 1657).

85. This digression was first noted and analyzed by Charles Webster, "The College of Physicians: 'Solomon's House' in Commonwealth England," *Bull. Hist. Med.,* 1967, *41:* 393-412.

86. Charleton, *Immortality of the Human Soul,* p. 35.

87. Ibid., pp. 35-37.

88. Ibid., pp. 183-85.

89. Walter Charleton, *Two Discourses. I. Concerning the Different Wits of Men: II. Of the Mysterie of Vintners* (London, 1669), pp. 50-51.

90. Harvey treated Anne Conway for headaches in 1651-1653. She corresponded with More, and mentioned Harvey to him in a letter of 26 January 1652/3. See Keynes, *Harvey,* pp. 392-95. More dedicated books to both Viscount Conway and Lady Conway during the 1650s.

91. Henry More, *The Immortality of the Soul* (London, 1659), p. 456.

92. Wallace Shugg, Walter Sherwin and Jay Freyman, "Henry More's 'Circulatio Sanguinis': An unexamined poem in praise of Harvey," *Bull. Hist. Med.,* 1972, *46:* 180-89. Shugg gives (pp. 185-86) several reasons for believing that the poem was written ca. 1651-1653. These are suggestive, but I would argue that More's works of the 1650s treat physiological questions, especially those concerning the heart and lungs, in such an unsophisticated way that he could not possibly have read *De motu cordis* at that time (Henry More, *An Antidote Against Atheism*

2nd ed., [London, 1655], pp. 142-57, especially p. 146; *Enthusiasmus Triumphatus* [London, 1656], passim; *The Immortality of the Soul* [London, 1659], pp. 157, 188-91, 208-14, 218, 270).

93. Shugg et al., ibid., pp. 185-186.

94. Thomas Fuller, *The History of the Worthies of England* (London, 1662), under "Kent," pp. 79-80.

95. Edward Chamberlayne, *Angliae Notitia: Or, The Present State of England: Together with Divers Reflections upon the Antient State thereof. The Second Part* (London, 1671), p. 458.

96. Thomas Hobbes, *Elementorum philosophiae sectio prima de corpore* (London, 1655), in "Epistola dedicatoria" to the Earl of Devonshire, dated 23 April 1655, sig. A2v.

97. Shugg et al., "Henry More's 'Circulatio Sanguinis,' " p. 185.

98. James Harrington, *The Common-Wealth of Oceana* (London, 1656), p. 2.

99. Matthew Wren, *Considerations on Mr. Harrington's Common-Wealth of Oceana* (London, 1657), p. 9.

100. James Harrington, *The Prerogative of Popular Government* (London, 1658), pp. 9, 21. Matthew Wren, *Monarchy Asserted or the State of Monarchicall & Popular Government in Vindication of the Considerations Upon Mr. Harrington's Oceana* (London, 1659), pp. 16-17.

101. Harrington, *Prerogatives of Popular Government*, sig. Alr.

102. For a calendar of Boyle's references to Harvey, see Richard A. Hunter and Ida Macalpine, "William Harvey and Robert Boyle," *Notes Rec. R. Soc. Lond.*, 1958, *13:* 115-27.

103. Robert Boyle, *Some Considerations Touching the Usefulnesse of Experimental Naturall Philosophy* (Oxford, 1663), First Part, p. 19. The essays in this Part are, both from Boyle's testimony and from internal evidence, datable to the period 1648-1654.

104. Robert Boyle, *Occasional Reflections upon Several Subjects* (London, 1665), Section II, p. 194. This "reflection" is datable ca. 1649.

105. Boyle, *Usefulnesse of Experimental Naturall Philosophy*, First Part, p. 55; Second Part, p. 223.

106. Ibid., First Part, p. 35; Second Part, pp. 72-73, 231.

107. Ibid., First Part, p. 5.

108. Ibid., First Part, pp. 93-94.

109. Ibid., First Part, pp. 54-55.

110. Ibid., First Part, p. 95.

111. Robert Boyle, *Some Motives and Incentives to the Love of God* (London, 1659), p. 56. This work was finished in 1648.

112. Boyle, *Usefulnesse of Experimental Naturall Philosophy*, First Part, pp. 35-36. Boyle elaborated on the story of the valves in *A Disquisition about the Final Causes of Natural Things* (London, 1688).

113. Charleton, *Darknes of Atheism*, sig. c2r.

114. Hobbes, *Elementorum philosophiae*, sig. A2v.

115. Abraham Cowley, *A Proposition for the Advancement of Experimental Philosophy* (London, 1661), pp. 23-24.

116. John Dryden, *"To my Honour'd Friend, Dr. Charleton, on his learned and useful Works,"* in Walter Charleton, *Chorea gigantum* (London, 1663), sig. b2r-v.

117. Joseph Glanvill, *Plus Ultra: Or, The Progress and Advancement of Knowledge Since the Days of Aristotle* (London, 1668), p. 14.

118. Ibid., p. 15.

119. Ibid., pp. 15-16.

120. Ibid., pp. 16-17.

121. Llewellyn (or Llewellin, Lluelyn, Lluellyn) was at Christ Church, Oxford, 1636-1648, M.D. 1653; he became a Candidate of the College of Physicians in 1653, and a Fellow in 1659. See Joseph Foster (ed.), *Alumni Oxoniensis: The Members of the University of Oxford,*

1500-1714 (Oxford: Parker, 1891) III, 921, and Munk, *Roll.* I, pp. 293-94. On Llewellyn's friendship with Cartwright and Berkenhead, see Martin Llewellyn, "To the rich Memory of my Honoured Friend the Learned Author," in Cartwright, *Comedies. Tragi-Comedies.* sig. [*16r-17v].

122. M[artin] Ll[ewellyn], "To the Incomparable Dr. Harvey, On his Books of the *Motion* of the *Heart* and *Blood.* And of the *Generation* of *Animals.*" in William Harvey, *Anatomical Exercitations. Concerning the Generation of Living Creatures* (London, 1653), sig. alv-2r.

123. Ibid., sig. a2r.

124. Ibid., sig. a2v.

125. Ibid., sig. a2v-3r.

126. Ibid., sig. a34-v.

127. On Collop, see F.N.L. Poynter, "An unnoticed contemporary English poem in praise of Harvey and its author, John Collop, M.D.," *J. Hist. Med.,* 1956, *11:* 374-83; and Conrad Hilberry, "Medical poems from John Collop's *Poesis Rediviva* (1656)," ibid., pp. 384-411. See also Conrad Hilberry (ed.), *The Poems of John Collop* (Madison: University of Wisconsin Press, 1962), pp. 3-30.

128. John Collop, *Poesis Rediviva: or. Poesies Reviv'd* (London, 1656).

129. Ibid., pp. 46-50, 52, 56-59.

130. Ibid., p. 57.

131. Ibid., pp. 57-58.

132. Ibid., pp. 52, 59.

133. Ibid., pp. 46-47.

134. Ibid., p. 50.

135. For an excellent introduction to the early phase of these attacks, see P.M. Rattansi, "The Helmontian-Galenist controversy in Restoration England," *Ambix,* 1964, *12:* 1-23.

136. [Marchamont Nedham], *Medela Medicinae. A Plea for the Free Profession and a Renovation of the Art of Physick* (London, 1665).

137. See Henry Thomas, "The Society of Chemical Physitians: An echo of the Great Plague of London, 1665," in E.A. Underwood, ed., *Science, Medicine and History* (London: Oxford University Press, 1953), II, pp. 56-71.

138. [Christopher Merrett], *A Letter Concerning the Present State of Physick* (London, 1665), pp. 14, 64.

139. Nathaniel Hodges, *Vindiciae Medicinae & Medicorum: Or an Apology for the Profession and Professors of Physick* (London, 1665), pp. 94-95.

140. [Timothy Clarke], *Some Papers Writ in the Year 1664. In Answer to a Letter Concerning the Practice of Physick in England* (London, 1670), p. 23.

141. Ibid., pp. 24-30.

142. Robert Sprackling, *Medela Ignorantiae: Or a Just and Plain Vindication of Hippocrates and Galen from the Groundless Imputations of M.N.* (London, 1665), p. 50.

143. George Castle, *The Chymical Galenist: A Treatise Wherein the Practise of the Ancients is Reconcil'd to the New Discoveries in the Theory of Physick* (London, 1667), p. 5.

144. Clarke, *Some Papers Writ in the Year 1664.* p. 16.

145. Castle, *The Chymical Galenist.* pp. 3-4.

146. [Daniel Cox], *A Discourse. Wherein the Interest of the Patient in Reference to Physick and Physicians is Soberly Debated* (London, 1669), pp. 89-90.

147. Ibid., p. 252.

148. Nedham, *Medela Medicinae.* p. 17.

149. Sprackling, *Medela Ignorantiae.* pp. 120-21.

150. John Twysden, *Medicina Veterum Vindicata: Or an Answer to a Book. Entituled Medela Medicinae* (London, 1666), pp. 29-30.

151. Ibid., pp. 30-31.

152. Ibid., pp. 31-32.
153. Castle, *The Chymical Galenist*, p. 4.
154. Christopher Merrett, *A Short Reply to the Postscript, &c. of H.S.* (London, 1670), p. 26.
155. Ibid., p. 42.
156. Nedham, *Medela Medicinae*, pp. 2, 11-19, 44, 48-49, 95, 237, 253, 258-60, 263-68, 381-82.
157. Ibid., pp. 11-19.
158. Ibid., p. 2; see also pp. 258-59.
159. See my forthcoming short article, "John Twysden on Harvey, Aristotle, and the blood."
160. Twysden, *Medicina Veterum Vindicata*, p. 9.
161. Ibid., p. 10.
162. Ibid., pp. 46-54.
163. Ibid., p. 47.
164. For a biographical sketch, see Humphry Rolleston, "Charles Goodall, M.D., F.R.C.P.: A defender of the Royal College of Physicians of London," *Ann. Med. Hist.*, 1940, 2: 1-9.
165. Charles Goodall, *The Colledge of Physicians Vindicated, and the True State of Physick in this Nation Faithfully Represented* (London, 1676), pp. 65-115.
166. Ibid., pp. 66-68.
167. Ibid., pp. 71-84.
168. Ibid., pp. 85-104.
169. Ibid., p. 86.
170. Ibid., pp. 86-91.
171. Ibid., pp. 105-15.
172. Charles Goodall, *The Royal College of Physicians of London Founded and Established by Law* (London, 1684), sig. Pp2r-Xx2v.
173. Ibid., sig. Rr2r-Ss3v.
174. Ibid., sig. Ss4r-Xx1r.
175. Joseph Glanvill, *Plus Ultra*, p. 15.
176. Henry Stubbe, *The Plus Ultra Reduced to a Non Plus* (London, 1670), title page.
177. Ibid., pp. 77-94.
178. Ibid., p. 78.
179. Ibid., p. 79.
180. Ibid., pp. 94-98.
181. Ibid., pp. 100-2.
182. Ibid., pp. 102-4.
183. Ibid., pp. 103-11.
184. Ibid., pp. 111-12.
185. Ibid., p. 112.
186. Ibid.
187. Ibid., p. 113.
188. Ibid., pp. 113-14.
189. Ibid., p. 114.
190. Joseph Glanvill, *A Praefatory Answer to Mr. Henry Stubbe, The Doctor of Warwick* (London, 1671), pp. 183-85.
191. Ibid., p. 185.
192. Ibid., p. 184.
193. Ibid., pp. 183-84.
194. [Gideon Harvey], *The Accomplisht Physician, the Honest Apothecary, and the Skilful Chyrurgeon, Detecting Their Necessary Connexion, and Dependence on Each Other* (London, 1670) adopts a stance for the regular practitioner, and against empirics, practicing apothecaries

and prescribing surgeons. The book is sometimes ascribed to Christopher Merrett, but internal evidence and later references make clear that it was written by Gideon Harvey.

195. Gideon Harvey, *The Disease of London: Or a New Discovery of the Scorvey* (London, 1675), sig. A4r.

196. Ibid., sigs. A4r-5r, pp. 129-44.

197. Ibid., p. 206.

198. Charles Mohun, 3rd Baron Mohun of Okehampton, who suffered a rapier wound 17 November 1676 while serving as a second to Lord Cavendish, and died 29 September 1677.

199. Gideon Harvey, *Casus Medico-Chirurgicus: Or, A Most Memorable Case of a Noble-man Deceased* (London, 1678).

200. Ibid., pp. 9-10, 20-22, 40-41, 70-71.

201. Gideon Harvey, *The Conclave of Physicians, Detecting Their Intrigues, Frauds, and Plots, Against Their Patients* (London, 1683).

202. Ibid., "Introduction."

203. Ibid., p. 28.

204. Ibid., p. 31.

205. Ibid., p. 23.

206. Ibid., p. 197.

207. Gideon Harvey, *The Art of Curing Diseases by Expectation* (London, 1689), pp. 177-78.

208. Ibid., p. 179.

209. Ibid., pp. 179-82.

210. Ibid., pp. 183-84.

211. [Thomas Guidott], *Gideon's Fleece: Or the Sieur de Frisk. An Heroick Poem. Written on the Cursory Perusal of a Late Book, Call'd The Conclave of Physicians* (London, 1684).

212. Ibid., p. 1.

213. Ibid., pp. 7-13.

214. Ibid., p. 11.

Index

Abundance of blood, 55, 61, 64, 65, 74-76, 79, 99 nn. 223, 228, 230, 100 n. 242

Albertini, Hannibal, 53-54, 55

Alchemy, 13, 14, 18, 20

Alcmaeon of Croton, 37

Allestree, Richard, 113

Alpinus, Prosper, 122

Analogical reasoning, 15-23

Analogies, mechanical. *See* Mechanical analogies in physiology

Anastomoses, arterio-venous, 47-51, 58-59, 63, 72; and the circulation, 79-81, 89, 100 nn. 248, 249, 101 n. 250

Anatomical authors: English, 105-9; in Harveian Library, 115

Anatomical Physician, the, 104, 107, 129-33, 135

Anatomists: ancient, 31-32, 46; English, 105-9, 113, 118, 120, 122, 124-35; Italian, 21, 76, 113, 130; Paduan, 62; Renaissance, 1

Anatomy: ancient, 31-32, 38; British (*see* English anatomical research); and clinical medicine, 31-32, 57, 105, 112, 126-28, 132-33, 135; College of Physicians defended by, 104, 125-26, 128-29, 131-32, 135-36; comparative, 21, 31, 33, 117-18; defended, 133; deprecated, 31-32, 104, 126, 129, 132-33; functional inference from, 31, 38-39, 45, 59, 61, 78, 100 n. 241; and natural theology, 121; pathological, 33, 66-67, 69, 86-87, 98 n. 198

Anaxagoras, 15

Ancients and Moderns, Harvey in the dispute over, 103, 112, 121-23, 125, 127-32, 135, 136

Animal spirits, 20. *See also* Spirits (physiological)

Animals, blooded and bloodless, 65, 66

Animism, 15-16, 17, 19, 22

Anthony, Francis, 7, 11-12, 14, 17-18, 23, 24 n. 11, 26 nn. 64, 65

Anthony, John, 3, 24 n. 11

Apothecaries, 4, 5, 7, 8-13, 24 n. 14, 25 nn. 27, 28, 124, 132, 142 n. 194. *See also* Society of Apothecaries, the

Argenterio, Giovanni, 52-53, 95 n. 121

Aristotelianism, 15, 22

Aristotelians, 130

Aristotle, 15, 16, 31, 32, 65, 121, 122, 127-28, 129, 130

Arterial blood, flux and reflux of, 49-51, 58, 61-62, 76, 100 n. 237

Arteries: contain blood, 45, 46-51, 79-80; functions of, 44-51, 59-90 passim; structure of, 62, 71, 75, 98 n. 217. *See also* Pulse, arterial

Arteriotomy, 46-51, 58-59, 72; and the circulation, 78-80, 82, 100 n. 247

Arundel, Earl of, 10

Astrology, 8

Astronomy, 115, 120, 136

Atomism, 15, 22, 27 n. 88

Attorney-General, the, 9

Attraction, 38, 39, 44, 48, 54, 67, 68, 70, 71; by heat, 36, 39, 42, 43, 61, 68, 70, 71-72, 86, 98 n. 213; by ligatures, 57-58, 70, 98 n. 213; by pain, 39, 40, 57, 58, 68, 70, 98 n. 213; by vacuum, 47-51, 68, 98 n. 213

Aubrey, John, 108, 113-14

Aurum potabile. See Gold, medicinal use of

Azygos vein, the, 56-57

Bacon, Sir Francis, 11, 20, 116, 122, 126, 136

Balance of trade, the, 27 n. 84

Barber-Surgeons' Company, 3, 4, 5, 9

Baroque period, the, 23

Bartholin, Thomas, 126

Baskerville, Simon, 10

Bathurst, George, 111

Bathurst, Ralph, 105, 111, 112, 113, 120, 138 n. 38

Bauhin, Caspar, 115

Berkenhead, Sir John, 117, 134

Bills of Mortality, 2

Biology, 15, 19, 22. *See also* Harvey, William, biological investigations of

Blood: functions of, 18, 110; impetus of, 63, 69, 71, 72, 79, 85; as nutriment, 38-39, 42, 44, 45, 47, 55-57, 60, 62, 65-66, 77, 85; origin of, 110, 111; as vehicle of heat and spirits, 52-53, 59, 62, 65-66, 68-69, 84-85, 110, 112, 124. *See also* Abundance of blood; Movement of the blood; Primacy of the blood; Sanguification; Whole of the blood

Bloodletting. *See* Arteriotomy; Venesection

Stephens, Philip, 105, 112
Stoics, the, 40
Streaking of blood in veins, 61, 82, 96 n. 161
Stubbe, Henry, 113, 127, 129-31
Succus nervosus, 128, 130
Suffocation from concentration of blood, 41, 42, 54, 55, 60, 64; Harvey on, 67, 69, 73, 86-87
Sun, relation of, to heart, 18-19
Surgeons, 3, 4, 5, 7, 9, 11, 12-13, 44, 57, 143 n. 194. *See also* Barber-Surgeons' Company
Surgery and vivisection, 32, 44
Swelling: causes of, 36, 39, 42, 52, 60, 64, 96 n. 160; Harvey on, 67-68, 70-72, 75, 83, 88; of veins, under ligation (*see* Ligatures, moderate, and the circulation)
Symbolism, 16-19
Sympathy, 40
Syncope. *See* Fainting
Systole. *See* Heartbeat, the

Technology, 19-22
Teleology, 22, 31, 50, 53, 75, 78, 99 n. 229, 100 n. 241
Temkin, Owsei, 90 n. 1
Tenant, John, 8
Tension. *See* Tonic motion
Terne, Christopher, 105
Thales, 16
Theological works, Harvey and circulation in, 117-18, 121
Therapeutics, 4, 8-9, 11-14, 17, 23, 28, 30, 35-38, 42-44, 48, 51, 55-59, 64, 67, 126, 128, 131. *See also* Movement of the blood, the, therapeutic manipulation of; Physiology in relation to pathology and therapeutics
Things natural, the, 29
Thomson, George, 135
Thoracic duct, the, 112
Thorax, the, 55-57, 65, 68
Thorius, Raphael, 3, 24 n. 13
Tonic motion, 17, 40-42, 52, 54, 93 n. 66, 95 nn. 120, 121; and the circulation, 83-86
Tonos, 93 n. 66. *See also* Tonic motion
Tourniquet, the, 44
Tower, Richard, 105
Turner, John, 11
Twysden, John, 126-28, 134

Unlicensed practitioners, 3-8, 11, 12; education of, 6-8, 12

Vacuum. *See* Attraction, by vacuum
Valves, mechanical, 21

Valves of heart, 59, 71, 74, 98, n. 219; and the circulation, 112, 121; and quantitative reasoning, 76-77, 78, 100 n. 242
Valves of veins, 63, 130; and the circulation, 80, 85-86, 89, 100 n. 240, 119, 140 n. 112; Fabricius on, 60-62, 130, 96 n. 156; Harvey's early views on, 71-72, 73, 75, 88, 98 n. 219
Variability. *See* Functions, variability of
Varicose veins, 60, 82
Veins: and the circulation, 82-83; nutritive function of (*see* Venous blood, outward flow of); other functions of, 44-46, 59-60, 66, 71-72, 97 n. 183; structure of, 71-72. *See also* Valves of veins
Venesection: in ancient medicine, 36-37, 43, 46, 50; and the circulation, 81-82, 89, 131; in Renaissance medicine, 51, 52, 55-57, 58-59, 61, 63, 64
Venesection controversy, the, 55-57
Venous blood, outward flow of, 38-39, 45, 47, 55-57, 60-62, 64; Harvey's views on, 64, 66, 72, 81, 82, 86, 97 n. 183
Vernon, Francis, 117
Vesalius, Andreas, 34, 55-57, 115
Vesling, Johannes, 112
Vital spirits, 18, 110
Vivification, 62; Harvey on, 65, 66, 68, 69, 72, 85
Vivisection, 34; in antiquity, 31, 32; Galen's use of, 44-46, 49-51; Harvey's use of, 68, 72, 74, 78-80, 89, 123, 136; Power's use of, 111; Spieghel's use of, 62; Warner's use of, 21
Vivisectional distortion, problem of, 32, 45-47, 48-49, 50-51, 61, 91 n. 22; in Harvey's work, 33, 72, 74, 78-80, 82, 88-89

Wale, Jan van der, 111
Wallis, John, 107, 110, 111
Ward, Seth, 112
Warner, Walter, 20, 21, 27 n. 83
Weapon-salve, the, 9, 19
Webster, Charles, 84, 113
Webster, John, 112
Wharton, Thomas, 105, 114, 122, 125, 126, 128, 132, 134
Wheat, relation of, to heart, 18-19
Whistler, Daniel, 105, 116
Whitteridge, Gweneth, 97 n. 174, 99 nn. 221, 230, 100 n. 242
Whole of the blood, 49-51, 53, 54, 60, 66, 67, 78-79, 81
Willis, Thomas, 105, 113, 120, 122, 126, 127, 128, 129, 130, 132, 133, 134
Wilson, Edmund, 116